W9-BNW-522

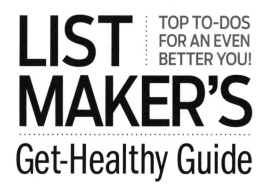

LIST
MAKER'S

TOP TO-DOS
FOR AN EVEN
BETTER YOU!

Get-Healthy Guide

LIST
MAKER'S

TOP TO-DOS FOR AN EVEN BETTER YOU!

Get-Healthy Guide

From the Editors of Prevention.

RODALE

This book is intended as a reference volume only, not as a medical manual.
The information presented here is designed to help you make informed decisions about
your health. It is not intended as a substitute for any treatment that may have
been prescribed by your doctor. If you suspect that you have a medical
problem, we urge you to seek competent medical care.

Mention of specific companies, organizations, or authorities
in this book does not imply endorsement by the author or publisher, nor does
mention of specific companies, organizations, or authorities imply that
they endorse this book, its author, or the publisher.

Internet addresses and telephone numbers given in this book
were accurate at the time it went to press.

© 2010 by Rodale Inc.

All rights reserved. No part of this publication may be reproduced
or transmitted in any form or by any means, electronic or mechanical,
including photocopying, recording, or any other information storage and
retrieval system, without the written permission of the publisher.

Rodale books may be purchased for business or promotional use
or for special sales. For information, please write to:
Special Markets Department, Rodale, Inc., 733 Third Avenue, New York, NY 10017

Prevention® is a registered trademark of Rodale Inc.

Printed in the United States of America

Rodale Inc. makes every effort to use acid-free ♾, recycled paper ♻.

Book design by Jenelle Wagner

Contributing writers: Elizabeth Shimer Bowers, Sandra Salera-Lloyd, Joely Johnson Mork,
Wyatt Myers, Maureen Sangiorgio, and Marie Suszynski

Pages vi, viii(3), ix(3), x, 7, 19, 28, 34, 43, 46, 51, 57, 66, 71, 73, 76, 79, 89, 92, 99, 103, 111, 117,
123, 127, 130, 141, 145, 150, 152, 155, 161, 167, 169, 173, 176, 182, 185, 189, 191, 195, 198, 201,
205: © Getty Images. Pages vii (7), 5, 11, 31, 41, 113, 137: © iStockphoto; Page 17: © Ted
Morrison; page 25: © Con Poulos; page 55: © Beth Bischoff; page 61, © Rubberball;
page 85: © Peter Lamastro; page 106: © Svend Lindbaek; page 115: © Deborah Jaffe;
page 118: © eStock Photo; page 133: © Ericka McConnell

Library of Congress Cataloging-in-Publication Data

List maker's get-healthy guide : top to-dos for an even better you! / from the Editors of
Prevention®.
    p.   cm.
    ISBN-13 978–1–60529–409–4 pbk
    ISBN-10 1–60529–409–8 pbk
    1. Health.   2. Hygiene.   3. Self-care, Health.   I. Prevention (Emmaus, Pa.)
RA776.9.L57   2010
613—dc22   2010019439

Distributed to the trade by Macmillan

2 4 6 8 10 9 7 5 3 1 paperback

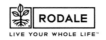

RODALE
LIVE YOUR WHOLE LIFE™

We inspire and enable people to improve their lives and the world around them.

To your best health

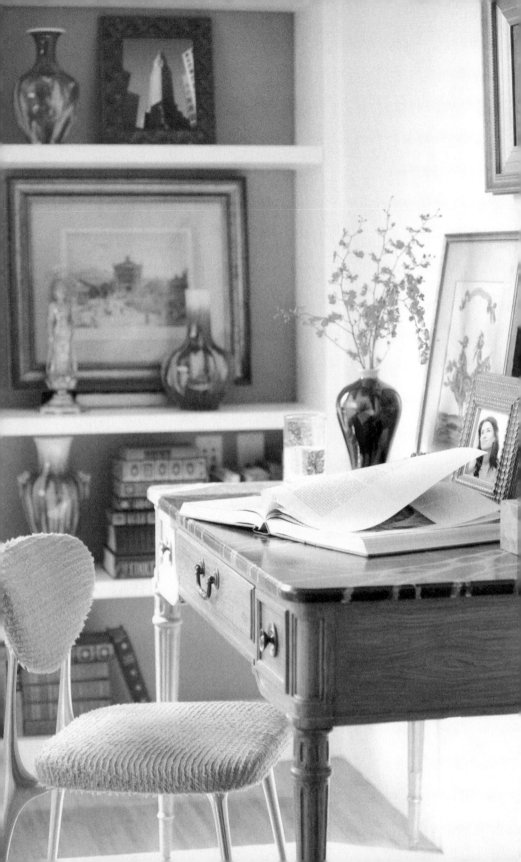

contents

introduction

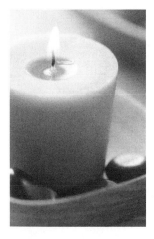 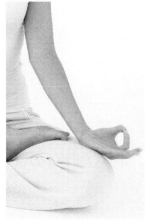 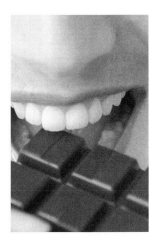

THIS IS A book of lists, so we can't think of a better way to lead off than with one. So here, then, are our top 5 reasons that a list is the perfect tool for helping you to shape and maintain a healthy lifestyle—however you define it.

1 A LIST GIVES YOU JUST THE FACTS

The universe of health information is constantly growing and evolving. That's a good thing, because it means that we're getting better at understanding how we can keep ourselves fit, healthy, and vibrant. The downside is that, as consumers, we can become overwhelmed by the dos and don'ts—especially when what was good for us last month, last week, or even yesterday suddenly turns out to be very, very bad (and vice versa).

With a list, we can weed out the distracters and focus on what's real and proven. As you read this book, some of the information may be familiar, which means that it's stood the test of time. But much of it is brand new, reflecting the latest science and expert thinking on a host of popular topics, from buying organic (page 12) to creating the perfect skin-care regimen (page 94) to getting a good night's sleep (page 146).

2 A LIST OFFERS CHOICES

Our nation's collective waistline seems to be growing in direct proportion to the number of diet plans and products on the market. This is true, at least in part, because no one dietary aid will work for everyone. We all have distinct genetics, family histories, personal preferences, and lifestyles. So we each need a self-care plan, whether we want to lose weight, lower our disease risk, manage stress, or improve our mental sharpness.

The beauty of a list is that you get to decide how much (or how little) you want to do in pursuit of a particular personal goal, based on the options presented to you. Pick your favorite advice from each list—or, for a challenge, see if you can use every tip in a list at least once. Try a few strategies and you'll discover which lists (and their components) work the best for you. Then use what you've learned to build a self-care plan that you can live with.

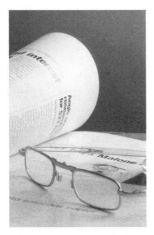 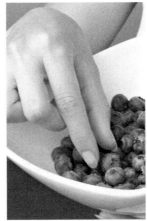 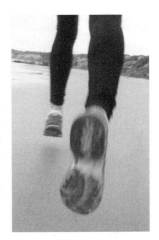

3 A LIST FEEDS A SENSE OF ACCOMPLISHMENT

Most of us keep a to-do list of some sort, whether it's scribbled on a Post-it or keyed into a PDA. And nothing feels as good as being able to cross off an item. It's visible proof we've achieved something.

Some days, just making a critical phone call or remembering to pick up the kids at soccer practice is a minor triumph. We can benefit from applying this same philosophy to a healthy lifestyle.

By parsing our big-picture goals into bite-size bits, we begin to make them doable. Going back to our weight-loss example, the prospect of losing 20 pounds may be daunting. But incorporating a serving or two of fat-fighting foods into your daily meals and snacks—now that seems easy enough, doesn't it? Likewise, doing *everything* experts recommend to be eco-friendly can be both impractical and expensive. But just washing laundry with cold water is an easy change that adds up!

4 A LIST IS FUN

From year-end best- and worst-ofs, to seasonal sports rankings, to the nightly Top 10, lists entertain as well as they inform. In navigating this book, no doubt you'll turn to the topics most relevant to you first. But we do encourage you to read the rest of the lists when you have a chance. You're guaranteed to find a few delights and surprises—not to mention some fascinating facts that might help break the ice at your next business meeting or dinner party. (Did you know, for example, that 53% of women spend more time trying to tame frizzy hair than they do exercising? Really!)

5 A LIST IS FINITE

It doesn't demand a long-term commitment or up-front resources. You can read a list, glean from it what's appropriate for you, and then move on to the next one. In this book, you've got 96 lists to choose from, on the topics that we at *Prevention* know best.

. . . .

We've had a blast crafting this collection just for you, in collaboration with a team of experts at the forefront of their respective specialties. Read the lists, absorb them, make them work for you. We think you'll agree: These lists make a healthy lifestyle as easy as 1, 2, 3!

—The Editors of *Prevention*

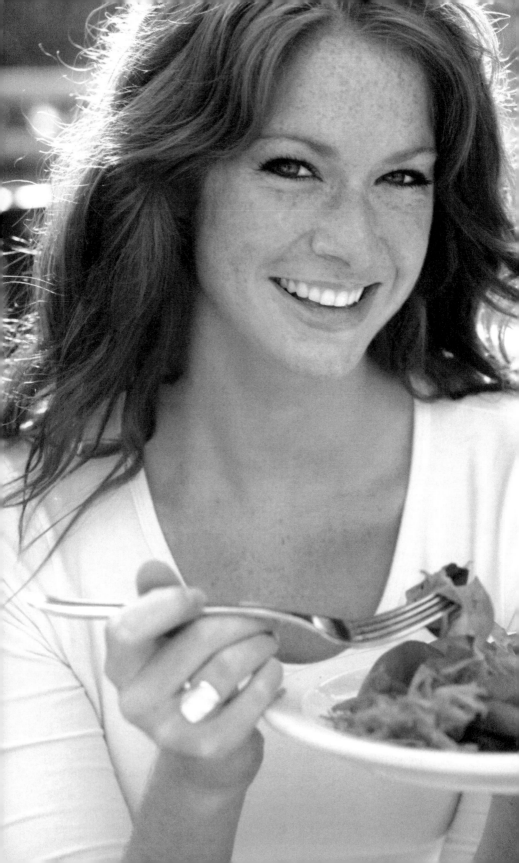

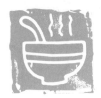

chapter 1 food

top 10 superfoods

facts & figures

50

percent

The number of "vegetables" in kids' diets that are actually french fries, according to a study from Ohio State University.

WHILE ALL FRESH, whole foods have something to offer nutrition-wise, the 10 chosen for this list are especially noteworthy for their nutrient profiles. They may not be regulars on your dinner plate now, but consider that the simple act of broadening your food horizons can measurably improve your health. Colorado State University nutritionists asked 106 women to eat 8 to 10 servings of fruits and vegetables daily for 8 weeks. Women who chose from 18 different varieties of produce reduced their rates of DNA oxidation, possibly making their bodies more resilient against disease, while those who ate the same 5 over and over again showed no change.

So don't be afraid to mix it up at mealtime! These top picks are a good place to start.

1 FRESH FIGS

Six fresh figs supply 891 milligrams of blood pressure–lowering potassium, nearly 20% of the recommended daily intake. In a 5-year study from the Netherlands, high-potassium diets were linked with lower rates of death from all causes in healthy adults age 55 and older. A serving of figs also has nearly as much calcium as ½ cup of fat-free milk!

Shop for figs that are dry on the surface. Chop and add to yogurt, cottage cheese, or green salads, or cut open and stuff with a low-fat soft cheese.

2 TURNIPS

One-half cup of this old-fashioned root vegetable has only 18 calories but is rich in cancer-fighting compounds called glucosinolates. Blend or mash boiled turnips into your favorite mashed potato recipe for a lower-calorie, high-nutrient comfort food.

3 LYCHEE

Among all of the fruits tested for a French study, which appeared in the *Journal of Nutrition*, lychee had the second-highest level of heart-healthy polyphenols—nearly 15% more than the amount in grapes.

Serve lychee by peeling the outer covering; use a knife to remove the pit. Add to stir-fries or kebabs for a sweet, grapelike flavor.

4 SPINACH

This leafy green is rich in lutein and zeaxanthin, carotenoids that help stave off age-related macular degeneration as well as cataracts. What's more, the vitamin K in spinach is essential for blood clotting and bone health, while the B vitamins (especially folate) help promote heart health.

5 ASIAN PEARS

One large Asian pear has nearly 10 grams of cholesterol-lowering fiber, about 40% of the recommended daily intake. According to one recent study, people who ate the most fiber had the lowest levels of total and "bad" LDL cholesterol. They also weighed the least and had the lowest body mass index and waist circumference.

Choose firm pears with a fragrant aroma and blemish-free skin. Dice into salads or make a flavorful dessert by simmering 2 large peeled, cored, and quartered pears with 1 cup white wine, 1 teaspoon honey, 1 teaspoon grated fresh ginger, and enough water to cover.

6 BOK CHOY

The glucosinolates in bok choy appear to be responsible for the potent anti-cancer properties of this vegetable. When it is cut or chewed, the glucosinolates get converted into isothiocyanates and indoles, compounds that in studies were able to inhibit or prevent tumor formation.

7 PAPAYA

Papaya is one of the top sources of beta-cryptoxanthin, which research suggests can protect against lung cancer. It also is rich in lycopene and contains the enzyme papain, which aids digestion. "Papain helps break down amino acids, the building blocks of protein," says Elisa Zied, RD, a spokesperson for the American Dietetic Association.

When shopping for papaya, choose a fruit with golden yellow skin that yields to gentle pressure. Cut lengthwise and discard the black seeds. Scoop out the flesh using a spoon and sprinkle with lemon juice.

8 SOY

Eating whole soy foods—such as tofu, soy nuts, and edamame (whole soy beans)—instead of high-fat proteins like steak and pork chops can reduce saturated fat and boost fiber in your diet. Soy protein may also help prevent the accumulation of belly fat in postmenopausal women, according to a study from the University of Alabama at Birmingham.

9 WILD SALMON

Salmon is packed with the omega-3 fatty acid DHA, a major component of neurons. People with the highest blood levels of this mega-nutrient are 47% less likely to develop dementia, according to a study published in the *Archives of Neurology*. Choose wild salmon over farmed; the latter doesn't always contain high amounts of omega-3s.

10 WALNUTS

A diet rich in walnuts may be more effective than the traditional Mediterranean diet at lowering levels of LDL cholesterol and lipoprotein(a), a compound that increases blood clotting and can lead to stroke, according to a study published in *Annals of Internal Medicine*.

your list

7 staples for your pantry

TAKING CONTROL OF what you eat begins with taking control of what you buy. By stocking up on a variety of nutrient-dense packaged foods, like the ones in this list, you always have the makings of a good-for-you meal at your fingertips. Because these foods don't spoil as quickly as fresh, they can help save a little on your grocery bills, too.

Just one caveat: With certain canned goods, sodium can be on the high side. Be sure to read labels and choose low-sodium products whenever possible.

mini LIST

A pair of pantry healers

When chapped skin or nighttime coughs strike, try turning to your kitchen cupboard instead of the medicine cabinet for relief.

1. **Oatmeal.** Researchers recently identified the avenanthramides in oats as the key compounds that calm inflamed skin. Put whole oats in a clean sock and seal with a rubber band. Drop into a warm bath, then climb in and soak for 15 minutes.

2. **Buckwheat honey.** When researchers from Penn State College of Medicine gave 105 children with coughs 1 to 2 teaspoons of buckwheat honey, cough medicine, or nothing before bed, those taking honey coughed less and slept more. For adults, try up to 3 teaspoons every 2 hours as needed. Don't give honey of any kind to children younger than 1 year.

1 CHICKPEAS

In a recent study, adults who ate 3 cups of chickpeas (also known as garbanzo beans, or *ceci* in Italian) a week cut both total and "bad" LDL cholesterol by 7 points. Try cooking up crunchy chickpeas: Rinse and dry canned chickpeas, spray lightly with oil, dust with spices, and bake at 350°F until golden brown.

Other varieties of canned beans make great healthy staples, too, so check out what's available at your supermarket.

2 BEETS

The antioxidant betanin in canned or pickled beets may protect against cancer and heart disease. Try a colorful beet, walnut, and greens salad: Top baby arugula (or other tender greens) with sliced beets, then sprinkle with goat cheese, walnuts, and balsamic vinaigrette.

3 CANNED WILD SALMON

Canned salmon contains heart-healthy omega-3 fatty acids, plus a generous dose of calcium from the tiny bones. It also has fewer pollutants (like PCBs) than farmed salmon. Make a light and easy salmon salad by blending 1 15.5 oz can of salmon, 2 tablespoons olive oil, 1 tablespoon lemon juice, and dried dill and capers to taste. Use it as a filling for sandwiches and wraps, or serve on a bed of greens.

Other kinds of canned fish, including tuna and sardines, are excellent protein choices. By all means stock up!

4 ARTICHOKE HEARTS

These exotic little vegetable bites contain inulin, a prebiotic fiber that boosts gut health and may help control appetite. Try a Mediterranean artichoke omelet: Sauté garlic, drained artichokes, and spinach for the omelet filling; top with a bit of crumbled feta and oregano. Save the flavorful liquid from marinated artichoke hearts (sold in jars) to drizzle onto green salads or grainy breads.

5 NUTS

USDA researchers have cracked the secret to a younger brain. Simply adding about seven to nine whole nuts to your daily diet may improve balance, coordination, and memory, finds new research published in the *British Journal of Nutrition*. The scientists believe that the polyphenols and other antioxidants in nuts such as walnuts help strengthen neural connections and improve cognitive skills. In addition, people who consume nuts more than four times a week have a 37% lower risk of heart disease. Add a handful to hot or cold cereals, salads, and even casseroles.

6 WHOLE-GRAIN PASTA

Spaghetti is a simple, filling comfort food, but noodles made with white flour tend to come up short on fiber, among other nutrients. These days, 100% whole-wheat pastas are widely available. If you or other family members are skittish about eating "brown noodles," ease the transition by first trying a lighter multigrain blend. Even these provide 4 grams of fiber per serving, compared with the 2 grams in "enriched" pasta.

7 BOTTLED PASTA SAUCE

No need to keep an entire inventory of different tomato products on the shelf. Bottled tomato sauce not only can top a plate of pasta, it also can stand in for canned or pureed tomatoes in other recipes. Be sure to choose a sauce in a glass bottle, which doesn't require a potentially hazardous resin lining. Several brands, like Trader Joe's and Pomi, are sold in food-safe Tetra Pak boxes.

If you are using pasta sauce as a substitute for canned tomatoes, the sauce should have few or no added ingredients. Otherwise, you may need to adjust your recipe to accommodate the already seasoned sauce.

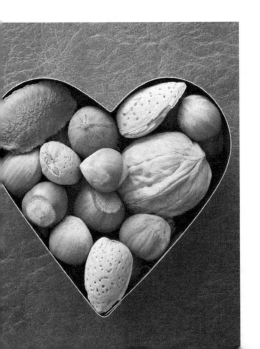

your list

5 must-haves for your freezer

mini LIST

Picking and preparing frozen produce

Frozen foods are a great convenience. These tips will help you turn them into great meals, too.

1. **Choose Grade A.** The Grade A designation means that the produce was carefully selected for color, tenderness, and condition. Grades usually appear on the back of the package, inside a symbol that looks like a shield.

2. **Skip sauces and salt.** When sauces are included, fat, sodium, and sugar levels typically skyrocket. The healthiest frozen food choices contain zero additives.

3. **Top with flavor.** Jarred tapenades or pestos are flavorful and coat veggies perfectly; most add a mere 40 calories and almost no sodium. Steam your favorite frozen vegetable, and toss with 1 tablespoon per cup of vegetables.

A LOT OF people think that fresh fruits and veggies are best, but believe it or not, frozen produce is even more nutrient-packed. That's because the moment fruits and veggies are harvested, they start to lose nutrients. Freezing slows that loss. A 2007 study found that the vitamin C content of broccoli plummeted 56% in 7 days when fresh, but dipped just 10% in a year's time when frozen at -4°F (-20°C). In addition, levels of disease-fighting antioxidants called anthocyanins and some minerals, including potassium, actually increased after freezing.

According to the Centers for Disease Control and Prevention, you should be eating about 2 cups of fruit and 2½ cups of veggies every day (1 cup is about the size of a baseball). Fortunately, hitting the mark is easier than you may think. Just 12 frozen baby carrots equal a cup, and with no chopping required, they're ready for nibbling in no time. From freezer to fork, most veggie side dishes or fruity desserts take less than 10 minutes to prepare. Here are some frozen staples to stock up on.

1 BLUEBERRIES

When researchers at Cornell University tested 25 fruits for antioxidant activity, they found that tangy-sweet wild blueberries (which are smaller than their cultivated cousins) packed the most absorbable antioxidants. Their levels exceeded those of nutrient-rich pomegranates and grapes. Look for frozen brands like Dole and Wyman & Sons. Defrost briefly before tossing into salads or mixing with ½ cup of low-fat ricotta and a drizzle of honey.

2 FRESH HERBS

You can have fresh, flavorful herbs all year round, and right at your fingertips. Wash and finely chop herbs such as parsley, oregano, and sage. Fill sections of an ice cube tray about halfway with herb pieces. Cover the herbs with water and freeze until solid. Pop the cubes from their trays, transfer to an airtight container (like a zip-close plastic bag), and store in the freezer. You can add the frozen cubes directly to the pot while preparing hot soups, stews, and sauces.

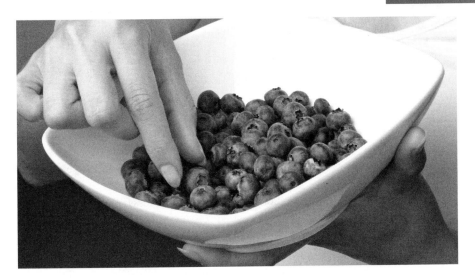

3 BROCCOLI

Though it's available year-round, broccoli is a cool-weather crop that is at its peak between January and March. Fresh broccoli should be used within a few days of purchase, but when frozen, it's available anytime. Choose loose-pack (bagged) rather than block (boxed) broccoli to make recipe measuring easier. Add frozen broccoli to marinara sauces, casseroles, and even omelets.

4 GREEN PEAS

Peas benefit from freezing because their essential sugars are captured right after harvest, before turning to starch. Look for frozen baby or petite peas, which have the best flavor. Toss still-frozen peas directly into soups or sauces for a colorful protein and fiber boost. Peas are also a good source of folate.

5 MIXED VEGETABLES

For an ultra-fast, delicious dinner, stir-fry a nutrient-packed vegetable blend with a protein of your choice (try tofu or beans for a vegetarian meal). Mixed veggies (California blend, for example) deliver a variety of colors, flavors, and nutrients, all in one convenient bag.

your list

7 foods that fight belly fat

mini LIST

Beat a "stress belly"

Anxiety increases levels of the stress hormone cortisol, a powerful biological trigger for weight gain. Here's how to stop it—fast.

1. **Eat slowly and pay attention to feelings of fullness.** This may lower cortisol levels and help decrease the amount of food you eat.

2. **Next time you're under duress, choose decaf.** When you combine stress with caffeine, it raises cortisol levels more than stress alone.

3. **Get enough shut-eye.** This may be the most effective stress-reduction strategy of all. A University of Chicago study found that averaging only 6½ hours of sleep each night can increase cortisol, appetite, and weight gain. The National Sleep Foundation recommends 7 to 9 hours.

VISCERAL FAT (BELLY fat) collects deep in your abdomen, around your internal organs. Because it's stored underneath your muscle layer, it doesn't jiggle. Instead, it swells your middle and gives you a round body shape, like an apple.

Some amount of fat is necessary to survive—to store fuel, protect our organs, and insulate us from the cold. But too much belly fat is a big health threat. It interferes with insulin production and blood sugar regulation, raises levels of "bad" LDL cholesterol, and secretes cytokines, which trigger the chronic inflammation that contributes to heart disease and type 2 diabetes.

Omega-6 fatty acids are the main polyunsaturated fat in the adipose tissue that makes up the belly fat of every overweight American. You can trim this fat by eating a healthy balance of essential fats—including beneficial omega-3 fatty acids—but not too many omega-6s at every meal.

A big belly also may be a side effect of sluggish digestion, leading to constipation and bloating, which can distend your belly beyond your waistband. High-fiber food choices can help move things along and leave your belly a bit flatter.

Bottom line: The larger your middle, the higher your disease risk. That means belly fat is nothing to fool with. If you've got it, you want to get rid of it. Now. These foods can help.

1 GREENS

Leafy greens, along with legumes and potatoes, have a better balance of omega-3s to omega-6s than most seeds and grains (though whole grains have other fat-melting benefits, as we'll discuss shortly). Omega-3s occur in the leaves of plants as alpha-linolenic acid (ALA). When we consume plant foods, our bodies convert ALA into even more dynamic omega-3s: EPA and DHA.

2 LEAN PROTEINS

Cows raised on grass produce meat, milk, and cheese with many more omega-3s than their corn- and soy-fed counterparts. Chickens fed a diet rich in flax and greens produce eggs that are as high in EPA and DHA as many species of fish.

3 FISH

Moderate fish consumption is more beneficial in a diet that has fewer omega-6s, which compete with the belly-flattening omega-3s. Try to eat at least two fish-based meals per week. Fish oil supplements can also help.

4 WHOLE GRAINS

A study published in the *American Journal of Clinical Nutrition* found that dieters who ate five servings of whole grains every day for 12 weeks lost twice as much belly fat as those who ate refined carbohydrates. The researchers credit the higher fiber in whole grains for the significant reduction in belly fat. Swap out white bread, pasta, crackers, and flour for whole-wheat and other whole-grain varieties.

5 GREEN TEA

Study participants who drank up to 5 cups of green tea daily had greater exercise-induced declines in ab flab than those who didn't drink tea, according to research in the *Journal of Nutrition*. The study's authors theorize that the catechins in green tea stimulate the body's fight-or-flight response, making exercise burn fat more efficiently.

6 PROBIOTICS

These beneficial bacteria can flatten your belly by improving digestion and reducing constipation and bloating. According to research from the University of Turku in Finland, they also may cut belly fat by altering how you use and store energy. Try yogurt drinks, cottage cheese, and other dairy products that deliver a dose of probiotics in each serving. (Look for the phrase "live active cultures" on the label.)

7 BANANAS

Potassium-rich foods such as bananas help your body get rid of excess water weight, minimizing your middle. The extra fluid is present because the two main minerals that control the amount of water in your body—potassium and sodium—have gotten out of balance. When your sodium level is too high, your tissues hold on to fluid. You can restore your sodium-potassium equilibrium by increasing your potassium intake. As you rebalance your system, you'll flush out the extra sodium along with the water. Presto: less puffiness! Besides bananas, good food sources of potassium include potatoes, papayas, tomatoes, and oranges.

your list

7 foods that sabotage your diet

236
calories

The number of
extra calories that the
average person
consumes on week-
ends, compared to
weekdays, according
to researchers at the
Washington University
School of Medicine.
That extra noshing
would add up to
a 9-pound weight
gain over the course
of a year.

WE'VE FOLLOWED ALL of the weight-loss rules, trading our lunchtime burger and fries for a salad, cutting back on snack foods and sweets, choosing fat-free over full-fat whenever possible. So if we're doing everything right, why is the needle on the scale stuck—or worse, moving in the wrong direction?

Even when we have the best of intentions, something as simple as a healthy but oversize snack can make us gain weight rather than lose. But finding small ways to save just 100 calories a day can take off 10 pounds in a year. With help from a few nutrition experts, we've put together this list of red-flag foods and some simple strategies to keep them from undermining your weight-loss efforts.

1 PRE-MEASURED PACKS
Are 100-calorie snack packs a part of your stay-slim repertoire? As it turns out, these pre-portioned treats may do more harm than good. When researchers from the Netherlands gave TV-watching students either two large bags of potato chips or several portion-controlled ones, those with the smaller bags ate twice as many chips. If you find yourself reaching for a second 100-calorie bag, leave the empty pack in plain sight: Previous research has shown that people consume less food when they can see what they've already eaten.

2 "DIET" TREATS
Fat-free and sugar-free don't necessarily mean low-calorie. For example, one brand of reduced-fat chocolate chip cookie supplies 47 calories—just 6 less than a regular cookie. Plus, studies show that people who are overweight take in twice as many calories when they eat low-fat snacks rather than the regular versions. If you have a cookie craving, advises Katherine Brooking, RD, a New York City–based dietitian, go for the real thing—but limit yourself to 150 calories' worth.

3 LIQUID CALORIES
A couple of cups of cappuccino (each with 2 teaspoons of sugar) and a couple of cups of tea (each with

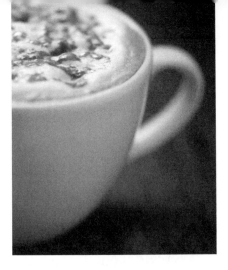

2 teaspoons of honey) add up to 150 calories in sweetener alone. Brooking recommends making do with less sweetener or switching to a zero-calorie alternative, like Splenda. Watch out for alcoholic beverages, too. Replace wine or beer with flavored club soda or sparkling water, and you can save big on calories.

4 SUPER-SNACKS

Eating every few hours is a good way to keep your metabolism humming, but it's easy to consume too many calories if you aren't careful. Snacks are the main culprits, particularly if they are too big and too frequent, explains Dawn Jackson Blatner, RD, author of The Flexitarian Diet. Limit yourself to just two snacks a day, at about 150 calories each. And be wary of relying on energy bars as snacks; some deliver as many as 400 calories each. As a rule of thumb, a bar under 200 calories is a snack, Blatner says; anything above that counts as a meal.

5 RICH PROTEINS

Stick with lean proteins because higher-fat versions can have twice as many calories. Even if you measure the proper serving size, just 3 ounces of sirloin supplies 225 calories, nearly half of which come from fat. By comparison, the same amount of skinless turkey contains 144 calories, only 10 of which come from fat. And turkey sausage has 75% less saturated fat than pork sausage. Other lean protein choices include fish and beans.

6 FAT-FREE SALAD DRESSINGS

Often the fat is replaced with sugar, which means that your dressing still may be loaded with calories. Ironically, a salad without fat is not living up to its potential. "You need a little fat to absorb vitamins A, D, E, and K and other nutrients," explains Katherine Tallmadge, RD, spokesperson for the American Dietetic Association. Instead, use smaller amounts of oil-based salad dressings; you'll get good-for-you fats rather than the saturated fat found in some creamy dressings. Look for ingredients like olive oil, vinegar, and herbs.

7 BAKED POTATO CHIPS

Yes, they're lower in fat. They're also high in calories but low in nutrients, with little fiber to fill you up. A better snack choice: popcorn. You'll get the salt and crunch of the chips in this whole grain, plus a healthy dose of fiber, all for about 65% fewer calories per cup. Look for oil-free microwave popcorn or brands that are air-popped or popped in healthful oils such as olive or canola. Adults who munch on popcorn consume up to 2½ times more whole grains than those who don't, according to a recent study published in the Journal of the American Dietetic Association.

your list ———
———
———
———
———
———
———
———

3 food groups worth buying organic

mini LIST

More ways to save on organics

Don't let cost stop you from benefitting from organic foods. These tips can help you make cost-effective organic choices.

1. **Go generic.** Many mainstream supermarkets now carry store-brand organics, including Safeway's O Organics line, H-E-B's Central Market Organic selections, Wal-Mart's Great Value private label, Stop & Shop's Nature's Promise, and Supervalu's Wild Harvest.

2. **Join a price club.** Money-saving organic options can be found at Costco, BJ's, and Sam's Club.

3. **Buy in bulk.** You can purchase many organic grains (including brown and wild rice and whole oats), pastas, flours, dried fruits, and nuts in the bulk sections of stores for far less. Organic brown rice is about 99 cents per pound in bulk.

WITH ALL OF the news about rising food costs, you may be wondering if the organic milk that you've been putting in your cart is worth the extra cash. It is. Organics may be more expensive, but for your dietary staples, they are a worthwhile investment. The benefits can positively affect your health not only today but long-term.

For a food to earn a USDA-certified organic seal, it must meet specific government standards. Organic meat, poultry, and dairy must come from animals that aren't given hormones or antibiotics, and organic crops are grown without using most conventional fertilizers, synthetic pesticides, or bioengineering. So what makes organic a better choice than conventional for certain foods?

Organics have more nutrients. Reports of organics not being better for you are outdated. An analysis of about 100 studies, including more than 40 published in the past 7 years, found that the average levels of nearly a dozen nutrients are 25% higher in organic produce.

Choosing organic may help you lose weight. Research involving laboratory rats found that those fed an all-organic diet (versus a conventional diet) had lower weights, less body fat, and stronger immune systems. Plus, the animals on a "clean diet" were calmer and slept better.

Going organic means avoiding toxins. Eating the 12 most contaminated fruits and vegetables exposes you to about 14 pesticides a day. A study supported by the EPA measured pesticide levels in children's urine before and after a switch to an organic diet. After just 5 days, the chemicals decreased to undetectable levels.

It isn't always easy to go organic, however. The number-one barrier to choosing organic produce over conventional is cost. By concentrating your organic purchases in a few core food categories, you can get the most benefit for your grocery dollar. Here's what we recommend.

1 FRUITS AND VEGETABLES

In the produce aisle, you may want to narrow your organic choices to those fruits and vegetables that tend to have the most pesticide residues in conventional form. Government laboratory tests show that even after washing, certain fruits and veggies carry much higher levels of pesticides than others.

Between 2000 and 2005, the not-for-profit Environmental Working Group (EWG) analyzed the results of nearly 51,000 tests of pesticide residues on produce. Based on the data, the EWG created a "dirty dozen" list of the most contaminated fruits and veggies. The top offenders include peaches, apples, bell peppers, celery, nectarines, strawberries, cherries, pears, grapes (imported), spinach, lettuce, and potatoes. For these foods, always buying organic is ideal. If that's too pricey, then focus on those "dirty dozen" fruits and veggies that you tend to eat most often.

2 MEAT AND POULTRY

A study published in the journal *Meat Science* compared the nutritional content of organic and nonorganic chicken meat. The researchers found that the organic samples contained 28% more omega-3s, the essential fatty acids that have been linked to reduced rates of heart disease, high blood pressure, type 2 diabetes, inflammation, depression, and Alzheimer's disease. Animals raised organically can't be given antibiotics or growth hormones.

The recommended portion for meat and poultry is 3 ounces, roughly equivalent to a deck of cards. You can save money on your organic purchases by sticking to this serving size and rounding out your meal with less expensive whole grains and veggies.

3 DAIRY

Per half-gallon, organic milk is more expensive than conventional—about $4 versus $2.50—but it's worth the splurge. Recent studies revealed that organic milk contains 75% more beta-carotene—about as much as in a serving of brussels sprouts.

Compared to conventional, organic dairy has 50% more vitamin E, a powerful antioxidant that supports the immune system and fights heart disease and cancer. It also contains 2 to 3 times more of the eye-friendly antioxidants lutein and zeaxanthin, and about 70% more omega-3s.

Like organic meat, organic dairy contains no hormones or antibiotics. Also, the feed given to dairy cows is pesticide-free. (In 2005, diphenylamine—a pesticide residue—was found in up to 92% of more than 700 conventional milk samples.) Current nutritional guidelines recommend three servings of dairy per day. Among the organic options, milk tends to be the most frugal choice at about 50 cents per 1-cup serving (versus 31 cents for conventional). Many organic dairy companies such as Stonyfield Farm (stonyfield.com) and Organic Valley (organicvalley.coop) offer printable coupons on their sites to help save money on their products.

your list

12 foods not worth buying organic

facts & figures

95 percent

The proportion of ingredients that must be organically produced in order for a food product to be labeled as "organic." The one exception to this is seafood; the USDA does not have standards for fish products, so an organic label on these foods means nothing.

STEP INTO ANY health food store, and you might feel as though you've stepped into an alternate universe: On those earthy-crunchy shelves, you're likely to find an organic version of just about everything, including cotton candy and chewing gum. While it's true that organic "junk foods" are better for the planet (possibly due to less packaging or more environmentally sound manufacturing processes), they generally aren't better for you.

Similarly, certain fruits and vegetables that are available in organic varieties may be just fine in their conventional form. A shopping guide created by the nonprofit Environmental Working Group (EWG) includes a list of the "clean 15"—the conventional produce selections that are lowest in pesticides and therefore OK to purchase.

The bottom line is that you needn't go organic across the board. Here are a dozen grocery items that you can confidently buy in conventional form.

1 SODA

A six-pack of organic soda can cost $5 or more. Yes, it's made without high-fructose corn syrup, but each can contains 160 calories (20 more than 12 ounces of Coca-Cola Classic) and zero nutrients.

2 LOW-CALORIE OR SUGAR-FREE ITEMS

If organic sugar-free cookies sound too good to be true, they probably are. Check the label for artificial sweeteners such as aspartame. If you're trying to keep it natural, you're better off choosing a nonorganic baked treat that's free of fake sugars.

3 SEAFOOD

Whether caught in the wild or farmed, fish can legally be labeled organic, even though it may contain contaminants such as mercury and PCBs, according to the Consumer Union, the nonprofit publisher of *Consumer Reports*. That's because the USDA has not yet developed organic certification standards for seafood.

4 ONIONS

These underground wonders rank lowest on the EWG's pesticide-load list. Stock up on conventional onions at the supermarket, and store them in a cool, dry place such as a pantry closet or low-humidity refrigerator drawer.

5 AVOCADOS

Fruits and vegetables that are peeled before eating generally deliver fewer pesticides, whether or not they're organic. For the record, and despite the thick skin, an avocado is a fruit—specifically a berry. Try ripe avocados, salt, and lime juice mashed together into savory guacamole.

6 CABBAGE

When tested by the EWG, more than 80% of cabbage samples showed no measurable pesticides. Shred raw cabbage into slaw or stuff steamed cabbage leaves with rice and bake.

7 FROZEN SWEET CORN

So much easier to prepare and enjoy than shucking niblets from the cob, and readily available year-round, conventional frozen corn is considered extremely low in pesticides. Use it in soups or cornbread mix.

8 FROZEN PEAS

Another freezer staple, peas are high in fiber and folate, two good reasons to have them on hand all the time. Choose baby or petite peas for tenderness and flavor.

9 TOMATOES

More than half of the tomatoes screened by the EWG contained no detectable pesticides, though they were most likely to have evidence of more than one kind of pesticide.

10 ASPARAGUS

Nearly all of the EWG's asparagus samples—90%—were pesticide-free. Lightly steamed or sautéed, asparagus lends a unique flavor as a side dish or ingredient.

11 PINEAPPLE

Fewer than 10% of the pineapple samples evaluated by the EWG were contaminated with any pesticides, and less than 1% had more then one kind of pesticide.

12 WATERMELON

Just over one-quarter of the EWG's samples showed evidence of pesticides. Ripe watermelons usually are a uniform color inside and shiny outside.

your list ———

———
———
———
———
———
———
———
———
———
———
———
———

6 best-for-you fast foods

facts & figures

52
calories

The number of
calories saved by
people who read
nutrition information
before ordering a meal
at a Subway restaurant,
according to a study
published in the
*American Journal of
Public Health*. Make
that choice (or a similar
one) every day, and
you could lose
5½ pounds over the
course of a year.

EATING AT WHAT many consider "healthy" fast food restaurants like Subway won't necessarily keep you as slim as Jared. Cornell University researchers recently stopped 500 diners as they left either Subway or McDonald's, asking them to estimate how many calories were in their meals. The average McDonald's patron guessed 876 calories when the real count was 1,093. By comparison, the typical Subway customer estimated 495 calories when the real count was 677—much higher than her guess!

"There's a big health halo that surrounds everything related to Subway," says Brian Wansink, PhD, lead researcher of the study and author of *Mindless Eating*. "People feel that they can justify extras like cookies and chips." What's more, when researchers tracked the diners at both fast-food establishments until dinnertime, the Subway group snacked more throughout the day, consuming an extra 112 calories, on average.

That said, there are healthy choices to be made at fast-food restaurants. The key word in that statement is "choices." Think before you order, and remember to say no to value meal deals that add extra items like fries and a drink. Odds are, any fast food add-ons will wind up doubling your calories with little to no extra nutrition.

1 FAT-FREE LATTE
At just 130 calories, you can get a dose of caffeine and a serving of healthy fat-free calcium with this afternoon coffee-shop treat. Just be sure to order a small, and if you'd like to add a little sweetness without doubling your calories, ask for a pump or two of sugar-free vanilla syrup.

2 CHILI
A small chili from Wendy's provides 227 calories, 5 grams of fiber, and a whopping 14 grams of protein. This hearty side is high in sodium (830 grams), but it also delivers 10% of a day's worth of iron.

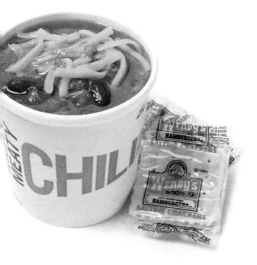

160- to 240-calorie Sammies, petite flatbread sandwiches like Sonoma Turkey and Bistro Steak Melt. Dunkin' Donuts has come out with Oven-Toasted Flatbread Sandwiches that are easy to hold and eat for breakfast or lunch. At less than 300 calories and about 6 grams of fat, these light meals are a guilt-free way to eat on the run.

6 GRILLED ITEMS

We're not talking burgers here. Usually, a fast food joint's grilled or roasted options—think turkey, chicken breast, lean ham, and even roast beef—provide fewer calories and less fat, according to experts at the Mayo Clinic. Skip the fries and be smart about the toppings (no mayo, more veggies), and you're on the right track.

3 LIGHTER FARE

A few chain restaurants have caught on to customers' cravings for lighter selections. For example, Au Bon Pain recently introduced a menu collection called Portions that features 14 dishes containing 200 calories or less, among them brie, fruit, and crackers; and chickpea and tomato salad.

4 BAKED POTATO

Even topped with chives and sour cream, a baked potato from Wendy's clocks in at under 350 calories, with 10 grams of protein and 8 grams of fiber. (A potato eaten with the skin is a top-notch source of fiber, as well as potassium.) You'll also get 110% of your daily vitamin C requirement, plus 20% of your recommended iron and calcium intakes—making this drive-through side a fairly well-rounded meal.

5 FLATBREAD SANDWICHES

Just because fast food is convenient doesn't mean it has to be oversized, fried, or served on a bun. Quiznos offers six

your list

6 worst-for-you fast foods

STUDIES SHOW THAT just hours after a person eats a typical fast-food lunch, fat globules start to collect in the blood vessels. It's easy to see why repeated consumption of these unhealthy meals can contribute to heart trouble, diabetes, and obesity. Blame this bad news on an overload of calories, fat, and sodium—the major concerns of a fast-food-heavy diet. All tie in to what may be the biggest (pun intended) problem with fast food: portion sizes.

The film *Super Size Me* shed light on megaportions—and not coincidentally, "supersize" options vanished from certain fast-food menus after the film's release. Still, oversized servings are the norm for the fast-food industry. McDonald's has unveiled a ⅓-pound Angus burger, which you can wash down with a 42-ounce beverage called a Hugo. That's roughly the equivalent of 477 calories of cola. Some establishments are being a bit sneakier: What was once a Great Biggie order of fries at Wendy's was reintroduced in 2006 as a large. It's 0.2 ounce smaller, but still in excess of 500 calories.

Best advice: When ordering fast food, choose the smallest size, regardless of its name. Stick with single-patty burgers, or order a kid's size. And be sure to steer clear of these foods if you want to keep your nutrition on track, even at the drive-through.

1 ARBY'S ROAST TURKEY & SWISS
Sure, it sounds healthy. But with those supersize slabs of bread, you get 725 calories, 8 grams of saturated fat, and more than a full day's worth of sodium! If you must, order it without the mayo to make it healthier, and save half of the sandwich for the next day.

2 SUBWAY FOOT-LONG SWEET ONION CHICKEN TERIYAKI SUB
Don't be fooled by the Subway "health halo." This sandwich delivers 9 grams of fat, not to mention nearly

mini LIST

A little light reading

Still hooked on fast food but want to make a change? Read about the real ins-and-outs of drive-through dining:

1. **Fast Food Nation:** *The Dark Side of the All-American Meal* by Eric Schlosser

2. **Eat This, Not That:** *Thousands of Simple Food Swaps That Can Save You 10, 20, 30 Pounds—or More!* by David Zinczenko with Matt Goulding

3. **Food Fight:** *The Inside Story of The Food Industry, America's Obesity Crisis, and What We Can Do About It* by Kelly Brownell and Katherine Battle Horgen

800 calories. On top of that, you'll be getting more than 2,000 milligrams of sodium with your sub. Most adults should consume less than 2,300 milligrams per day.

3 CINNABON CARAMEL PECANBON

At 1,100 calories, 141 grams of carbohydrate, 8 grams of protein, and 56 grams of fat (no, that isn't a typo), this sticky-sweet treat from the food court is more like a dirty and dangerous trick. Do yourself a favor and steer clear of this monster "snack."

4 MCDONALD'S FILET-O-FISH

Usually fish is a healthier choice than a burger, but not in this case. A McDonald's Filet-O-Fish contains 380 calories, which isn't that outrageous—until you consider the 18 grams of saturated fat. To make this sandwich less of an insult to your heart, ask for no mayonnaise or tartar sauce; at about 100 calories per tablespoon, these condiments can add up fast.

5 BURGER KING TENDER-CRISP CHICKEN SANDWICH

The Tendercrisp will fill you up with 800 calories and 46 grams of fat. Add a side and/or a soda to your sandwich, and you'll be getting way more than a full day's allotment of calories and fat in one sitting—without a single respectable serving of veggies or fruit in sight.

6 TACO BELL VOLCANO NACHOS

With a name like "volcano," you can expect the worst. And you won't be disappointed: Weighing in at 1,000 calories, 62 grams of fat, and 1,930 milligrams of sodium, this nacho "snack" has all the makings of a nutritional disaster. Its one redeeming quality is its 16 grams of fiber, a testament to the sheer volume of this volatile side dish.

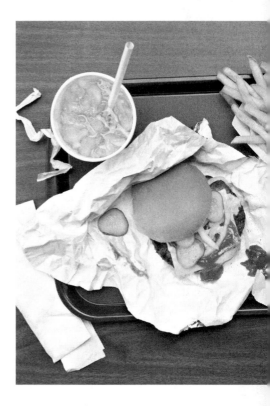

your list

7 smart strategies for dining out

my favorite...
Restaurant Survival Strategy

Alicia Fagan, an editor of medical journals from Wayne, Pennsylvania, uses this method to maintain her trim figure while traveling on the job.

Faced with a fancy menu that dares to dazzle you with choices that sound so delicious, are all diets off? Keep it simple, and stay focused, Alicia advises. "I seek out the most natural, whole-food ingredients that I can find on the menu," she says. "In the descriptions of dishes, I look for key words that identify leafy greens, vegetables, lean proteins, and whole grains. I'm wary of salads with a lot of fat and little nutrition (think, Caesar salad with croutons), and I avoid white starches like regular pasta and white rice."

EXPERTS AGREE THAT there's a correlation between expanding portion sizes and our expanding waistlines. And restaurants are known for dishing out way more food than we should be eating. According to a University of Minnesota study, people eat about 300 more calories at lunch when they're presented with large portions.

If you dine out often, pay attention to the portion sizes. Ask for a take-home container and pack up half of your food at the start of your meal, rather than waiting to see how much you can eat. Also, scan the menu for lighter entrées that deliver flavor, satisfaction, and nutrition without breaking the calorie bank. Here are more tips to help you choose wisely from any menu.

1 KNOW WHAT A PORTION LOOKS LIKE
A serving of meat, fish, or poultry is 3 ounces, approximately the size of a deck of cards or your palm. A serving of rice or pasta is ½ cup, or a mound about the size of a computer mouse. An actual pat of butter or a serving of salad dressing is only as big as your thumb tip. And a serving of cheese is 1 ounce, which looks like four dice cubes.

2 DO YOUR RESEARCH
If you've got a big dinner on your calendar, take some time to peruse the menu before you go. That way you can choose your meal more carefully—and you won't be tempted by the sight and smell of food while you wait to place your order. Many restaurants provide detailed menus on their websites; if not, call ahead and ask about the range of entrée options, so you won't be caught off guard.

3 BE INQUISITIVE
It's OK to ask questions about how a particular dish is prepared or if the chef would be able to skip the sauce. Don't be afraid to ask your server if substitutions are available for menu items.

4 DELAY THE BREAD
There's nothing wrong with enjoying the breadbasket, as long as you refrain from eating it all at once. Ask your server to bring the bread to your table at the same time as your main course. Or tell your server to skip the bread altogether. With good conversation, you'll hardly miss it.

5 DO THE BUFFET "BROWSE AND BOOTH"
Serve-yourself smorgasbords with their all-you-can-eat allure tend to be diet duds. But new research shows that there are fundamental differences between how overweight and healthy-weight people approach a restaurant spread. First, look before you eat: 71% of normal-weight diners—versus 33% of obese people—scanned the buffet's food selections before serving themselves. Then, request a booth: 38% of normal-weight diners sat in a booth instead of at a table, compared to 16% of obese people. When you sit in a booth, it isn't as convenient to get up and go for seconds.

6 GO FISHING
Even the most hard-core steakhouses can do a great job with seafood. Choosing a fish entrée is a great way to stay on track when dining out, according to the American Heart Association. In general, broiled or grilled fish dishes have fewer calories and far less fat than beef or pork. Some seafood choices, like tuna and wild-caught salmon, deliver added benefits in the form of heart and brain-friendly omega-3 fatty acids.

7 SHARE DESSERT
Just can't look past the dessert cart? It's okay to indulge once in a while. Again, portion size is critical: A 1-ounce serving of dessert—say, a brownie—is roughly the size of an average woman's thumb.

Turn dessert into a social event by ordering one and sharing it with your companions. Make sure that everyone gets his or her own fork!

your list

6 surprising health foods

mini LIST

What's in a health food?

According to experts at the Mayo Clinic, the healthiest foods meet at least three of the following criteria:

1. A good or excellent source of fiber, vitamins, minerals, and other nutrients

2. Rich in phytochemicals and antioxidant compounds such as vitamins A and E and beta-carotene

3. May help protect against heart disease and other medical conditions

4. Low calorie density, meaning that you get a larger portion for fewer calories

5. Widely available

IF THE LOW-CARB craze of the early 21st century left you believing that potatoes equal pounds and corn is no better than candy, it's time to wake up and taste the produce. The truth is, certain fruits and vegetables—along with other foods with less than stellar nutritional reputations—are rich in vitamins and minerals, not to mention an array of colors, flavors, and textures. If you've been avoiding the following dietary outcasts, it's time to give them another look.

1 POTATOES

For the 161 calories in a medium baked potato with skin, you get 4 grams of fiber plus 20% of your daily requirement for potassium, along with a boatload of phytochemicals known as kukoamines. Both potassium and kukoamines help keep your blood pressure in check. If you allow that cooked potato to chill before eating it, you'll get a generous dose of resistant starch, a fiber-like substance that promotes post-meal satiety—important for losing weight without feeling hungry.

"If you keep portion sizes in check—no more than one medium potato in a given meal—and eat the fiber-rich skin, potatoes make a satisfying, low-calorie, nutrient-rich side dish," says Michelle Dudash, RD, a Gilbert, Arizona–based dietitian.

2 ICEBERG LETTUCE

Just 1 cup of shredded iceberg lettuce delivers nearly 20% of your daily dose of vitamin K, a nutrient that many women don't get enough of. When Harvard University researchers tracked the diets of more than 72,000 women, those who ate one or more servings a day of any type of lettuce (all are good sources of vitamin K) had the lowest rates of hip fracture. Iceberg lettuce also is a good source of vitamin A, which helps keep your vision sharp; just 1 cup supplies 15% of your recommended daily intake. So if iceberg lettuce is the leafy green that floats your boat the most, go ahead and eat up!

3 CELERY

This pale, crunchy veggie delivers a unique combination of disease-fighting vitamins, minerals, and phytochemicals. For example, celery is a good source of pthalides, rare compounds that lower your blood pressure by relaxing artery walls. It also is rich in apigenin, a potent plant chemical that protects against cancer by inhibiting gene mutations. Munch on celery sticks for a low-calorie, crunchy snack: One large rib has just 10 calories and 1 gram of filling fiber.

4 CORN

Corn does double duty as a veggie and a whole grain, with one large ear supplying 15% of your recommended daily fiber intake. It also satisfies 10% of your daily folate requirement; this heart-healthy B vitamin plays an important role in keeping blood levels of potentially dangerous homocysteine in check. Not to be outdone, the lutein and zeaxanthin in corn help protect your eyes against age-related macular degeneration.

For a simple corn salsa, toss together fresh or thawed frozen corn kernels; finely chopped jalapeno chili pepper; chopped fresh cilantro, tomato, and onion; and a pinch each of chili powder or ground cumin.

5 WATERMELON

The amino acid arginine, abundant in watermelon, might promote weight loss, according to a new study in the *Journal of Nutrition*. When researchers supplemented the diets of obese mice with arginine over 3 months, the animals' body fat gains declined by a whopping 64%. Adding this amino acid to the diet enhanced fat and glucose oxidation while increasing lean muscle, which burns more calories than fat. Snack on watermelon while it's in season, and enjoy other arginine sources—such as seafood, nuts, and seeds—year-round.

6 BUTTERMILK

It might sound as rich as cream, but in fact, buttermilk has 98% less fat. This tart, thick dairy product contains beneficial bacteria that convert the milk protein lactose into lactic acid, a natural preservative. Buttermilk can be used in place of milk in many recipes, reducing fat and calories; it makes pancakes, waffles, and cakes rise quite nicely, and it adds a tangy flavor to smoothies and salad dressings.

your list

4 unhealthiest health foods

my favorite . . .
Strategy for Navigating Health-Food Stores

Mara Drogan, a graduate student from Troy, New York, follows this advice to avoid weight gain with her busy schedule.

When sorting out the unhealthy from the healthy at the local health-food store, the clues may be in the wrapping. "All those pre-packaged 'light' and 'healthy' meals seem more like robot food than people food to me," Mara says. "Anything that's highly processed or that can survive a nuclear winter can't be good to eat—no matter how many seductive words, like 'organic' and 'all natural,' appear on the label. Basically, if it's in a box with a bar code and it says 'homemade,' I know it isn't, and I don't buy it."

EVEN IF YOU haven't bought full-fat mayo or sugary soda since blue eye shadow was in style (the first time), you may be getting duped into less-than-stellar food choices at the supermarket. "From a distance, some foods seem like healthful choices because of the way they're packaged or labeled," says Janel Ovrut, MS, RD, a Boston–based dietitian. "But just because a product's marketing gives it an aura of health doesn't necessarily mean it's good for you."

Here is a short list of notorious health food impostors, plus smarter swaps that up the nutritional ante and still deliver the flavor you crave.

1 VEGGIE SNACKS

Have you taken up noshing on crunchy veggie snacks to up your produce intake? Bad move. These processed foods are high in fat, low in veggies. The truth lies in the ingredient lists. Potato flour, for example, lacks the robust nutritional profile of the unprocessed tuber. Tomato puree is a rich source of cancer-fighting lycopene, but these snacks contain only a modest amount. Fresh spinach and beets are loaded with nutrients, but the powdered form has little nutritional value. If you see canola oil in an ingredient list, it means that the snack is fried, supplying about the same amount of fat as regular potato chips. Not to mention that one serving of veggie snacks has nearly 300 milligrams of sodium.

For a healthier snack, try Organic Just Veggies. This crunchy mix uses whole peas, bell peppers, corn, tomatoes, and carrots. One serving has 100 calories, 1 gram of fat, 40 milligrams of sodium, 60% of the Daily Value for vitamin A, and 45% of the Daily Value for vitamin C. Visit justtomatoes.com to find a retailer near you.

2 ITEMS FROM THE HOT FOOD BAR

Freshly made doesn't equal healthy. For example, mashed potatoes prepared with butter, whole milk, and salt are fresh and unprocessed, but they can be high in saturated fat, cholesterol, and sodium. Even a cup of organic mac 'n' cheese can contain upward of 410 calories and 16 grams of fat (10 grams of it saturated).

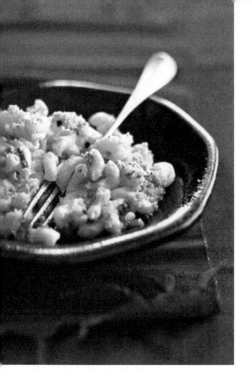

or white sugar, but they can be loaded with sugars in disguise, such as turbinado, Sucanat, and Florida sugar crystals. These are derived from sugarcane and beets, the same as refined sugars, so they're just as high in calories but without any extra nutritional value. For example, all-natural Sundrops contain more calories and cholesterol per gram than their conventional counterparts, M&M's. An oatmeal-raisin cookie by Alternative Baking Company, made with organic unrefined cane sugar, is egg- and cholesterol-free. But it still supplies a whopping 480 calories and 18 grams of fat.

Instead, buy cookies that are sweetened with fruit juice and lower in fat. Fabe's brand has 90 calories and only 4 grams of fat per serving (which equals 3 very small chocolate chip cookies). Choose oatmeal-raisin or peanut butter varieties for an extra nutrition kick. If portion control is a problem, buy one fresh bakery cookie instead of a store-bought box.

When lunching at the local hot food bar, look for potatoes with skins and dishes in which fruits and veggies are the primary ingredients. Also stop by the salad bar and load up on marinated vegetable and whole grain salads, olives, and cooked beans.

3 FAD FATS

They're bad by any name. Ghee, or clarified butter—promoted as a healing food in Ayurvedic medicine—doesn't deserve a healthy label. It contains the same amount of artery-clogging saturated fat as regular butter and was found to promote cardiovascular disease in four separate studies.

Also, beware of artisan cheeses and premium ice creams. They may be gourmet, but they're still high in calories and saturated fat. Stick with liquid vegetable oils, trans-free spreads, and low-fat cheeses, all found in abundance at these stores.

4 NATURAL SUGARS

It's true that "healthy" snack foods aren't made with high-fructose corn syrup

your list

_____
_____
_____
_____
_____
_____
_____
_____
_____
_____
_____

8 snacks to stash in your desk

facts & figures

$42 billion

Amount spent
by Americans on
vending machine
snacks in 2004. That's
a lot of quarters—and
a lot of calories.

WHEN YOU'RE AT home and the cupboards are stocked with healthy choices, it's fairly easy to eat well. What happens, though, when you're away from your own kitchen and you have less control over what's available to nibble on—like, say, when you're at work? If you're like a lot of people, you may find yourself being drawn to those classic dietary obstacles: boxed donuts, birthday cake, and candy bars and chips from the vending machine.

One way to reduce your chances of going overboard on calories is to stock your desk or lunchbox with delicious, nutritious treats. Ignore the call of certain snacks that may give you a quick spike in energy, only to leave you crashing from all the sugar and artificial additives.

The best workday snacks provide a mix of healthy complex carbohydrates, some healthy fats, and enough protein to provide energy and keep your metabolism and blood sugar levels on an even keel, advises Marissa Lippert, RD, owner of Nourish, a nutrition counseling and communications practice, and author of *The Cheater's Diet*. Here are her recommendations.

1 DRY CEREAL

A high-fiber cereal like Uncle Sam's, Kashi GoLean, or Heart to Heart is convenient to store and easy to eat dry, though you certainly can add milk if it's available in the company café. Find a cereal with at least 5 grams of fiber per serving, which will help keep your energy up, your blood sugar level stable, and your hunger at bay throughout the morning and afternoon.

2 TEA

It's 2 o'clock and you're starting to drag. Instead of heading for the coffee pot, brew yourself a cup of green or white tea, which has less caffeine. Or make a refreshing cup of peppermint tea, which has been shown to boost mental acuity and alertness. Keep a few tea bags in your stash, and just add water.

3 LOW-FAT POPCORN
Got a hankering for salty, crunchy goodness? Skip the chips and reach for a microwave-ready, low-fat popcorn like Newman's Own or Good Health. Besides satisfying your craving, you'll get a healthy dose of fiber. You'll even have enough to share, if you like.

4 NATURAL NUT BUTTER
Spread a tablespoon of natural peanut butter or almond butter on a couple of whole-grain crackers (such as Wasa, Finn Crisp, Kavli, or Dr. Kracker) or a slice of whole-grain bread (one that supplies at least 3 grams of fiber). For variety, try cashew or even sunflower butter. The combination of complex carbohydrate, protein, and healthy fat can give you the balanced energy you need to push through those last few hours of the day.

5 APPLE
Whether you slice it and spread it with peanut butter or eat it fresh out of hand, nothing beats a ripe, juicy apple as a day-brightening snack. Instead of hiding it in your desk drawer, put your apple—along with other fresh fruit—in a pretty bowl on your desk. You'll have a week's worth of healthy treats right at your fingertips.

6 NUTS
Roasted, unsalted nuts (think walnuts, almonds, pistachios, cashews, and pecans) are powerhouses of protein and healthy fat. Walnuts, in particular, are a good source of omega-3 fatty acids, known to boost brain health—just in time for that big presentation. Keep a bag of your favorite nuts on standby, or rotate through a selection.

7 LOW-CALORIE ENERGY BARS
Nothing beats an energy bar for convenience, but keep an eye on the fiber content (more is better) and calories (less is more). Try Kashi TLC granola bars, Gnu Flavor & Fiber bars, or Lara bars for a ready-when-you-are satisfying snack that delivers a dose of filling fiber for only around 200 calories each.

8 DARK CHOCOLATE
It's OK to indulge in a little chocolate—especially dark chocolate (70% cocoa or higher), which is packed with antioxidants. Besides satisfying your sweet tooth, it may lift your mood a bit, possibly because of its effect on serotonin (or just because it tastes so good!). A serving of chocolate does contain more calories than most of the other snacks mentioned here, so enjoy in small bites—think two or three small squares of dark chocolate. This is a case where quality definitely trumps quantity.

your list

6 tips to satisfy a sweet tooth

facts & figures

14
billion

Number of gallons of
soft drinks sold by US
beverage companies in
2008. That's 506
12-ounce servings for
every American adult
and child.

AS BABIES, WE have a natural aversion to bitter foods and a preference for sweets, says Jennifer Fisher, PhD, assistant professor of pediatrics at Baylor College of Medicine. While our palates become more sophisticated as we get older, many of us never lose our penchant for sugary foods. Scientists attribute our collective sweet tooth to the fact that so many poisonous plants are bitter. That is to say, preferring sweets has been critical to our survival as a species.

Candy-coveting also might be programmed into our DNA. New research has revealed that people with a certain variation of the gene glucose transporter type 2 (GLUT2), which may help the brain regulate food intake, are more likely to crave sugary foods.

We may never be able to explain why so many of us continue to fall under sugar's spell. But as Fisher observes, "What we do know is that sweet tastes better to us." That doesn't mean we must sacrifice nutrition for flavor. Why not satisfy your sweet tooth naturally? These tips can help you do just that.

1 REACH FOR SWEET VEGGIES
With their natural sweetness, yams, squash, peas, and carrots can help cure a sugar craving while still packing a nutritional punch. Raw red peppers are another satisfyingly sweet (and crunchy) snack.

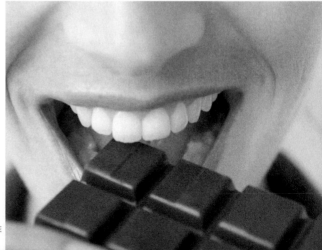

2 SNACK ON DARK CHOCOLATE

Dark chocolate may help you feel full, so you eat less, according to a new study from Denmark. Researchers there gave 16 participants 100 grams of dark or milk chocolate, followed by pizza 2 hours later. The people who consumed the dark chocolate ate 15% fewer calories than those who had the milk chocolate. The dark chocolate eaters also were less interested in fatty, salty, or sugary foods. Look for dark chocolate made with 70% or more cocoa. Two tablespoons of dark chocolate chips sprinkled over fresh berries can take the edge off of a sweet tooth without blowing your calorie budget.

3 MAKE YOUR OWN "SODA"

The average 12-ounce can of regular cola contains more than 150 calories but has zero nutritional value. Swap your pop for seltzer water flavored with juicy fresh-cut fruit such as ripe berries or citrus.

4 SPICE THINGS UP

Love breakfast cereal and home-cooked oatmeal—but only after spooning on table sugar or maple syrup? Use cinnamon, vanilla, clove, or nutmeg instead; you'll enjoy a big, calorie-free flavor boost and maybe reap extra health benefits besides. A study in the *Journal of Agriculture and Food Chemistry* found that among 30 plants tested, cinnamon and clove were among the highest in antioxidants. You also can add any of these spices to plain yogurt or steamed low-fat or fat-free milk.

5 POP SOME PEPPERMINT

Chewing on peppermint-flavored gum and drinking peppermint tea are two great options to quell a budding sugar binge. Researchers at Wheeling Jesuit University found that people who simply sniffed peppermint ate 23% fewer calories, on average, over a 5-day period.

6 BE FRUIT-FULL

Not all sugars are created equal. The two main classes are naturally occurring sugars (from Mother Nature) and added sugars (by food companies). Don't limit the former. Though an orange can contain 12 grams of sugar, it also provides vitamins, minerals, and antioxidants. Plus, the natural sugars in sweet produce don't raise diabetes risk in the same way that added sugars do. No health organization recommends limiting natural sugars, so keep filling your cart with sweet, colorful produce.

your list

4 ways to stop a salt craving

my favorite...
Cure for a Salt Craving

Alicia Fagan, an editor of medical journals in Wayne, Pennsylvania

For some people, a salt craving may be a good time to eat something green. "When I crave salt, I feel like my body is really telling me that it needs minerals," Alicia says. "I'll eat a big salad of greens and herbs (such as parsley and cilantro) or a few stalks of celery to help replenish other minerals."

Celery does contain a bit of salt (about 40 milligrams per medium stalk), but it's also a good source of a host of nutrients, including calcium, magnesium, manganese, phosphorus, potassium, B vitamins, and vitamins A, C, and K.

IF EVERYONE ATE just $\frac{1}{2}$ teaspoon less salt per day, it would prevent 750,000 new cases of heart disease and save more than half a million lives over a decade, according to new calculations by researchers at the University of California, San Francisco. Nearly 80% of the salt in our diets comes from processed foods such as breads, canned soups, and canned veggies. That excess sodium not only raises your heart disease risk, it also makes you retain water, puffing up your belly.

But cutting back on salt isn't easy. In addition to salt just plain tasting good, over time we grow accustomed to a certain level of saltiness, so less salty foods taste bland in comparison. New research suggests that salt may even deliver a mood-elevating effect. No wonder cutting back on sodium can be such a daunting, if worthwhile, task.

To shake the excess salt from your diet, start by limiting your consumption of processed foods such as canned soups and frozen entrées; they're responsible for up to 75% of the sodium in the typical American diet. Next, abstain from sprinkling extra salt onto your meals. Every seven to eight shakes adds another $\frac{1}{2}$ teaspoon.

Here are a few simple suggestions for satisfying a salt craving without adding a lot of extra sodium to your diet.

1 LOOK FOR "LOW SODIUM"

Big-name brands like Pepperidge Farm, Campbell's, and Del Monte are rolling out reduced-salt versions of old favorites such as chicken noodle soup and canned sweet peas, slashing sodium content by up to 50%. Many pasta sauces, canned and boxed broths, and dry soup mixes also are available in low-sodium varieties. Read product labels to make sure that you're not exceeding the recommended 2,300 milligrams of sodium per day.

2 SWITCH SHAKERS

You needn't overhaul your diet to reduce your sodium intake. Setting down the saltshaker may be enough. Scientists at Shiraz University in Iran asked 60 adults with high blood pressure to refrain from salting their foods and eating obviously salted snacks, such as potato chips and salted peanuts. After 6 weeks, the participants' systolic blood pressure declined by 8%, a drop that the researchers say cuts stroke risk by 33% and heart disease and heart failure by 25%.

Try sodium-free seasoning blends to add flavor without salt. You can even make your own: Combine equal amounts of three of your favorite savory herbs (try basil, oregano, and marjoram), plus the same amounts of garlic and onion powders. Use this aromatic mixture to replace the salt in your tabletop shaker.

3 PICK POTASSIUM-RICH FOODS

Potassium helps the kidneys excrete surplus sodium, which is especially important for regulating blood pressure. Adults need about 4,700 milligrams of potassium per day. To meet your requirement, load up on bananas and other potassium-packed foods: cooked corn, baked potatoes, kidney beans, ground flaxseed, papaya, quinoa, walnuts, raisins, and low-fat yogurt. (Note: If you're taking any blood pressure medication, check with your doctor before increasing your potassium intake.)

4 SNACK ON SOY NUTS

Here's a crunchy, salt-free snack that could slash blood pressure to boot. Postmenopausal women who replaced half of their daily protein with ½ cup of soy nuts reduced their systolic blood pressure by as much as 5.2% over 8 weeks. Those with hypertension saw even greater improvements: Their blood pressure declined up to twice as much, and their "bad" LDL cholesterol dropped by 11%.

To liven up the taste without adding many calories (there are 240 calories in ½ cup of plain soy nuts), toss the nuts in a zip-top bag, lightly spritz with cooking spray, and sprinkle with salt-free Cajun seasoning or apple pie spice. Shake and eat!

your list ———

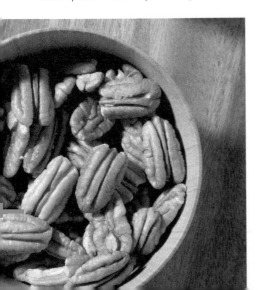

7 tips to sneak in more veggies

my favorite . . .
Way to Eat More Veggies

John Oravec is a husband and new father in Philadelphia, Pennsylvania, who is inspired to help keep his family healthy.

John says it's tough even getting grownups to eat their veggies. But he has a few tricks up his sleeve. "My wife has a problem with texture. She doesn't like anything crunchy or slimy, or things that have a skin or peel," John explains. "To sneak vegetables into pasta sauce, I just puree a blend of onions, garlic, carrots, zucchini, bell peppers, and eggplant right in with the fresh tomatoes. I cook all the vegetables together with some wine and olive oil, and then use a hand mixer or blender to whirl up the chunks into an acceptable smoothness. Delicious and healthy!"

WE DON'T NEED to tell you to eat more vegetables; there are only, oh, a few hundred health reasons to do so. Numerous studies link a higher veggie intake to reduced risk of cardiovascular disease, stroke, cancer, type 2 diabetes, and obesity. Every major health organization, including the American Heart Association, American Institute for Cancer Research, and American Diabetes Association, recommends eating a wide variety of vegetables on a daily basis.

Unfortunately, some of the chemicals that make veggies so healthy are the very ones that cause many of us (not just 5-year-olds) to shudder at the sight of steamed greens. In fact, as many as 30% of Americans are extra sensitive to the bitter taste of the chemicals in these vegetable; nutrition experts call these people supertasters.

For others, it isn't the taste but the lack thereof that makes them turn up their noses at vegetables. Many veggies pack a lot less flavor than they could, points out Tristan Millar, former director of marketing and business development for Frieda's, the specialty produce marketer in Los Angeles. "American growers have focused on varieties that ship well and spoil slowly. There's been little emphasis on taste."

But with a bit of extra know-how at the supermarket and in the kitchen, you can still reap the very real benefits of this essential food group. Use the following ideas to get more vegetables into your diet, starting with your next meal.

1 SUBSTITUTE SOUP

If you don't like the taste of many vegetables, soup may be your best solution. Most cook for so long that the vegetable flavors mellow and weaken, while the seasonings become more pronounced. Almost any kind of soup will do, providing you add a few cups of chopped fresh (or frozen) veggies—such as broccoli, peppers, cauliflower, and carrots—before simmering.

2 GET OUT THE GRATER

Mix grated carrots or zucchini into muffin batter, bread dough—even meat loaf. The next time you make a meat loaf, after adding the usual 1 cup of bread crumbs and 1 egg, throw in 1 cup of grated vegetables of your choosing. Onions, zucchini, mushrooms, and even green beans will be virtually undetectable. While the longer baking time breaks down some nutrients, most of the vitamins and minerals stay in the casserole. Plus, the veggies make for a moister meat loaf.

3 REPLACE MEAT WITH VEGGIES

In some dishes, cutting back on meat may allow you to "secretly" increase the veggie content. And yes, tomato sauce counts (½ cup equals one full serving of veggies). But why stop there? Try adding at least two other naturally nutrient-rich veggies to every dish. You'll bolster the flavor and the bulk—and enjoy a bigger serving size for very few extra calories.

4 BED 'EM BETTER

The next time you serve grilled chicken breast or broiled fish filets, present the classic meal over a bed of steamed corn kernels or lightly sautéed greens instead of rice. The veggies add color and texture to otherwise familiar fare—and they count toward your daily veggie quota.

5 RECONSIDER KALE

With its reputation for toughness, kale often is passed over. But it's rich in vitamins A, C, and K, not to mention an excellent source of calcium. What's more, eating cruciferous veggies like kale may lower your cancer risk. Try this simple recipe to turn kale into surprisingly delicious, crispy "chips" perfect for snacking: Chop kale and drizzle it with olive oil, salt, and pepper, then bake it at 350°F for about 15 minutes.

6 USE YOUR BEAN

Did you know that beans count as a vegetable as well as a protein source? Canned or dried, they add a blast of protein, vitamins, and fiber to any meal. Even better, they're easy to camouflage. The next time burgers are on the menu, try mixing cooked mashed beans and mushrooms with lean ground beef or turkey.

7 MAKE SUPER SLAW

Here's news that may pique your interest in a few raw veggie superstars: People who ate uncooked broccoli, cabbage, or cauliflower at least three times per month were 40% less likely to develop bladder cancer than those who ate the veggies less frequently, according to researchers at Roswell Park Cancer Institute in Buffalo, New York. Turbocharge a popular side dish by substituting Mann's Broccoli Cole Slaw (shredded broccoli, red cabbage, and carrots) for the usual amount of shredded cabbage in your favorite coleslaw recipe.

your list

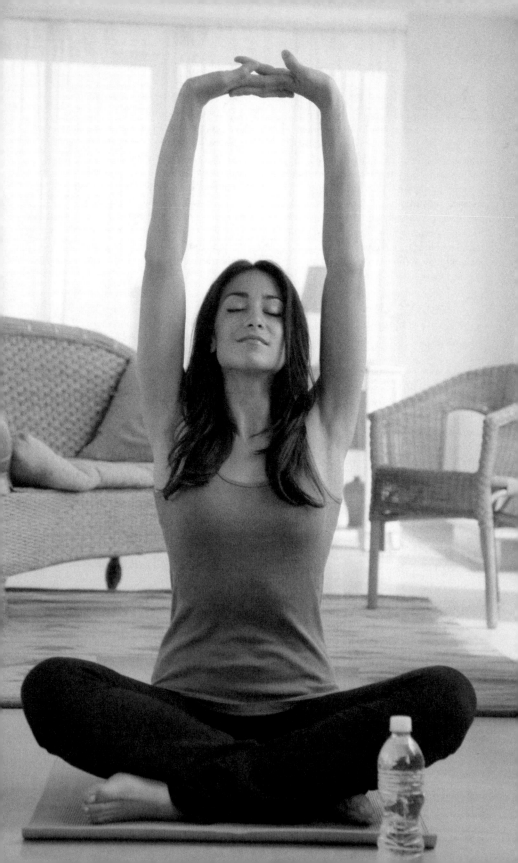

chapter 2 fitness

top 10 reasons to exercise

facts & figures

1,440 minutes

The number of minutes in a day. A good workout takes just 30 minutes, or 60 if weight loss is your goal.

ACCORDING TO A 2008 survey, there are more American adults who don't exercise than there are those who do. Of the people who responded, only 33% reported that they get their hearts pumping with regular physical activity.

The nonexercisers are missing out on a boatload of health benefits, from improving their mood to protecting themselves from disease. Take a look at the top 10 reasons why you should include yourself among the regular movers-and-shakers.

1 YOU'LL LOSE WEIGHT

It's this simple: You lose weight when you burn more calories than you take in. Cutting calories through dietary changes helps, but adding exercise to the mix can make an even bigger dent. Consider this: You burn a measly 80 calories while sitting on the couch watching an hour-long television show, but hop on a treadmill and walk at a 3-mile-an-hour pace, and you'll bump up your calorie burn to 320.

To lose weight, experts recommend working out at a moderate to vigorous pace for 60 minutes most days of the week. Just be careful not to overeat and gain your hard-lost calories back!

2 YOU'LL LOWER YOUR DISEASE RISK

Getting your heart pumping on a regular basis can help prevent heart disease, high blood pressure, high cholesterol, type 2 diabetes, osteoporosis, and some cancers. This protective effect is due at least in part to the fact that people who exercise tend to weigh less, says Vincent Perez, a physical therapist for Columbia Doctors Eastside in New York City.

3 YOU'LL BOOST YOUR IMMUNE FUNCTION

Regular exercise is among the trio of lifestyle factors that keep your immune system up and running, the other two being a healthy diet and reduced stress. Experts even say that a brisk walk for 20 to 30 minutes five days a week can have a bigger effect on your immune system than nutrition. Research also has suggested that working out regularly may cut by half the number of days that you're sick with a cold or the flu.

4 YOU'LL FEEL ENERGIZED

Getting in a workout increases the circulation of oxygen and nutrients throughout your body. That means your heart and blood vessels won't have to work as hard, leaving you with more energy throughout the day. Exercise also can help you get a good night's sleep, so you'll wake up rested and ready to go in the morning.

5 YOU'LL BE HAPPIER

Ever notice that you feel better after a workout than you did before? It's because physical activity stimulates chemicals in your brain that help you to relax while brightening your mood. Exercise also has been shown to protect against depression. In a large study of more than 14,000 people over 12 years, researchers found a lower incidence of depression among those with moderate to high fitness levels.

6 YOU'LL BE LESS STRESSED

Studies have shown that people who exercise have fewer health problems when they're under stress. It doesn't take much physical activity to do the trick. A Scottish study of 20,000 adults found that working out for just 20 minutes a week helped to lower stress and anxiety while increasing energy and happiness.

As a physical therapist, Perez has noticed that his patients are less bothered by stress after they exercise. He attributes this to the "feel-good" endorphins released during physical activity.

7 YOU'LL FEEL MORE CONFIDENT

Those endorphins also help you feel good about yourself, which can raise your confidence level. So does setting a fitness goal and accomplishing it, along with watching your body change and become leaner and stronger.

Becky Wenner, a certified personal trainer and owner of Becky's Fitness Company in Bayside, Queens, has a client who gained so much confidence after starting to exercise that she started her own business. Another client decided to leave her job and study to become a nutritionist, with the goal of eventually starting her own consulting service.

8 YOU'LL THINK CLEARER AND REMEMBER MORE

Recently researchers tracked 1,324 people who were participating in the Mayo Clinic Study of Aging. They found that those who were moderate exercisers at age 50 and older were less likely to develop mild cognitive impairment later in life.

9 YOU'LL HAVE BETTER SEX

Men who are active are at lower risk for developing erectile dysfunction than men who are inactive. Exercise can increase sexual arousal in women as well. When you're fit, you feel better about your body, and you have more energy for a romp in the sheets.

10 YOU'LL LIVE LONGER

All of those health benefits add up to a longer life. A study of more than 5,000 people found that those who were moderately active after age 50 lived one and a half years longer than those who were sedentary. People who were highly active lived 3½ years longer.

your list ──────

_____

_____

_____

_____

_____

best 10-minute workout

my favorite...
Fitness Move

Tara Zimliki, certified personal trainer

"This is an amazing exercise that gives you big results because it really works your legs," Zimliki says. "You do two fast jump lunges (alternating legs) followed by two jump squats. Then repeat the sequence. Beginners should aim for 18 repetitions, though when I have a full day of classes, I will do as many as nine sets of 18. I don't recommend doing this exercise more than once a week. Do it on a Friday (or the day before you're going to rest), so your body has time to recover before you work out again."

THINK YOU DON'T have enough time for a good workout? Before you skip it, ask yourself if you can spare just 10 minutes. That's all you need to work your major muscle groups and get your heart pumping, says Tara Zimliki, a certified personal trainer and owner of Tara's Bootcamp in Branchburg, New Jersey. Although she usually recommends exercising for 30 to 45 minutes 5 days a week, she says that a focused 10-minute workout can help make you stronger and burn calories.

For this workout, you'll need a pair of 3- to 5-pound hand weights. Watch the clock as you perform the following moves, completing as many of each as you can in 1 minute. If you have 20 or 30 minutes—even if it's split into 10-minute segments throughout the day—by all means, do two or three sets, Zimliki says.

1 WARM UP
Start by marching in place for 30 seconds and going into a light jog for 30 seconds, which will help rush blood to your muscles and get you ready to work out.

2 PUSH-UP WITH A SIDE PLANK
Do full push-ups with your hands a little wider than your shoulders and your legs straight behind you, or modified push-ups by keeping your knees bent and your ankles crossed. With your abs pulled in and your body in a straight line, lower yourself down and up.

After you come up from each push-up, do a side plank. Turn your body to lie on one side with your knees bent and one leg resting on top of the other. With your elbow under your shoulder, tighten your abs and push your hip off the floor, keeping your bottom knee on the floor, and hold for a second before releasing. Alternate sides after each push-up.

3 FRONT LUNGE WITH CHEST FLIES
With a 3- to 5-pound hand weight in each hand, step forward with one leg, bending at the knee. Drop your back leg down until your knee almost touches the ground. Be sure that the knee of your front leg doesn't go past your foot.

At the same time as you step into the lunge, lift your weights out to the sides with your palms facing forward. Then push back into a standing position as you press your hands forward to complete the chest fly. Alternate legs as you do the flies.

4 BACKWARD LUNGE WITH A TRICEPS KICKBACK

Still holding the hand weights, take a large step backward, dropping your back leg until your knee almost touches the floor. Make sure that your front knee doesn't go past your foot. Keep your arms bent and your elbows close to your body. As you come up from the lunge, straighten your arms behind you for a triceps kickback. Then return your arms to the starting position before lunging again.

5 SQUATS AND OVERHEAD SHOULDERS

Stand with your feet shoulder-width apart, holding the weights at your shoulders. Bend your knees and lower yourself until your thighs are parallel to the floor, as though you're about to sit in a chair. Make sure that your knees don't go past your feet. Then push through your heels and stand up, straightening your arms and clinking the weights together when they're above your head. Lower your arms back to shoulder height and repeat.

6 JUMP SQUATS

Without your weights, squat down and push yourself up into a jump, landing back on your feet before lowering into a squat again. To help keep your balance, Zimliki suggests holding your fists in front of you.

7 PLIE SQUATS

Stand with your legs a little farther than shoulder-width apart and your feet in a V position. Lower your butt toward the floor as you do for a regular squat, then explode up into a jump. Repeat.

8 THE PLANK

Lie facedown on the floor, then prop yourself on your toes and your elbows, keeping your body in a straight line from your ankles to your head and pulling your abdominal muscles as tight as possible. Hold this position for a full minute. (Going longer than that can put too much stress on your back, Zimliki says). If you can't stay in this position for 60 seconds, go as long as you can, then take a short break before repeating. Gradually work up to 1 minute straight.

9 JACKKNIFE

This is an advanced move, so Zimliki recommends doing it for 30 seconds rather than a full minute. Lie flat on your back, putting a small rolled-up towel under your lower back if necessary for support. Straighten your arms above your head and tighten your abdominal muscles. Then lift your arms and your legs at the same time, keeping them straight, and touch them where they meet above your body. Lower them and repeat.

To make it easier, keep your legs straight up in the air and move your arms toward your legs, Zimliki says.

10 COOL DOWN

With your legs shoulder-width apart, bend at your waist and reach down toward the ground. Touch the ground between your legs and hold for several seconds. Move your chest toward your right knee and hold, then toward your left knee and hold.

your list ———

————————————
————————————
————————————
————————————

8 must-have fitness tools

my favorite...
Exercise Equipment

Becky Wenner, certified personal trainer

Wenner recommends a resistance band because it is inexpensive and lightweight, and it can travel with you. "A good band will offer some resistance when you do a biceps curl but won't be so loose that the exercise is too easy," Wenner says. Here's how to test it: Stand on the band with your feet hip-width apart and your hands in the handles (or ends for bands without handles). With your arms on either side of you and your palms facing forward, lift them into a biceps curl. If the band is a good fit for a biceps curl, it should be a good length for all arm and leg exercises.

WHEN LIFE GETS hectic, you can't beat the convenience of working out at home. You may not have time to run to the gym or even head outdoors for a walk, but you can always hop on the treadmill first thing in the morning or lift hand weights while watching TV.

When you're thinking about purchasing fitness gear, keep in mind that a well-rounded exercise program includes tools that will assist with both aerobic activity and strength training. Here's what experts recommend having on hand, though the most important part of choosing exercise equipment is buying what you like and what you're most likely to use.

1 SHOES

Your first and best investment should be in a pair of sneakers that are appropriate for your activity, fit well, and provide good support. They'll help you avoid injury and increase your performance when you exercise, says Jari Love, a certified personal trainer in Calgary, Alberta, Canada, who created a workout program called Get Ripped! Some experts recommend replacing your shoes every 300 to 500 miles, but another good guideline for regular exercisers is to buy a new pair every three months or so, Love says.

2 PEDOMETER

The biggest advantage of a pedometer is that it measures your activity all day long, not just when you're on a treadmill or another piece of exercise equipment, says John P. McCarthy, PhD, associate professor in the department of physical therapy at the University of Alabama at Birmingham. It motivates you to stay active even in between workouts, as you think of ways to add to your daily step count.

3 HEART RATE MONITOR

Many treadmills have built-in heart rate monitors, so if you're buying a treadmill (which we'll discuss shortly), you may not need a separate heart-monitoring device. But if you're looking for something to keep tabs on your intensity level when you walk or jog outside, a portable model is the way to go.

Like a pedometer, a heart rate monitor can push you to work out harder, Love says. You'll end up getting a better workout because you'll be able to keep your intensity in a range that affords optimal benefits.

4 WEIGHTS

Strength training should be a component of everyone's exercise routine. But the type of weights you buy depends on personal preference.

If you have the room and the budget for a large piece of equipment, you can invest in a weight machine that will work all of your major muscle groups, McCarthy says. For a more economical option, choose hand weights. A number of companies now offer adjustable dumbbells that allow you to change the amount of weight with the flip of a switch, McCarthy says. This may be a better option than individual dumbbells; with these, you'll need to buy an entire set so that you have the right weight to work small muscles like your triceps as well as larger muscles like your chest.

5 IPOD OR MUSIC PLAYER

For some, listening to music is essential to getting through a workout. In fact, it may help you to work harder, Love

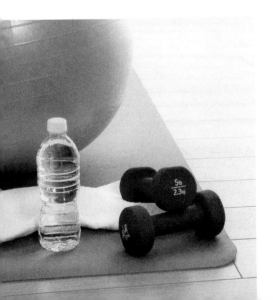

says. Research has shown that people exercise 30% longer when they're listening to high-intensity music.

6 TREADMILL

If you're willing to spend $700 to $1,000, consider investing in a treadmill. It's probably the most popular piece of equipment for aerobic activity, McCarthy says. With a treadmill, you can walk, jog, run, and do hills—all in the comfort of your own home.

McCarthy recommends a model that goes up to 8 miles per hour, with an incline of at least 10%. Some models offer preprogrammed workouts, which are great for mixing up your fitness routine.

Check for safety features, such as arm grips, side rails, and an emergency shut-off clip. Also, make sure that the track you'll be walking on isn't so narrow that you can easily step off the side and isn't so short that you don't have a safety cushion behind you if you slow down. Your best bet is to try out several treadmills in person before buying.

7 WEIGHT GLOVES

They'll protect your hands against calluses and give you more control over the weights, Love says.

8 STABILITY BALL

A ball is inexpensive and versatile. You can use it for abdominal exercises, as a substitute "bench" when you're lifting weights, and for strength exercises.

your list ——————

————————————————

————————————————

————————————————

————————————————

————————————————

4 crunchless belly flatteners

my favorite...
Core Exercise

Pete McCall, exercise physiologist

One of McCall's favorite core exercises uses a cable machine at the gym. Here's how to do it: Stand with your back to the machine, with a cable in each hand. Brace your abs and press one hand forward at shoulder level, pushing the cable away from you. The cable will make you feel as though you need to rotate your body; this is where your abs come into play, as they help keep your body facing straight ahead. Work up to two or three sets of 6 to 12 repetitions each.

WE CAN'T HELP but envy the flat, muscular abs that we see on magazine cover models. They must spend hours doing crunches to get so taut and toned, right?

Not necessarily. Some of the best moves for great abs have nothing to do with the familiar lift-and-tuck. "People are surprised that they can do an abdominal workout without crunches," agrees Pete McCall, an exercise physiologist and spokesman for the American Council on Exercise.

Your core muscles—those that surround your torso and pelvis—are designed to work most effectively when you're standing upright and moving, McCall explains. So it makes sense to get up off the floor to work your abs. Besides, if you have back trouble, crunches can aggravate the pain.

Here's how to get a flatter stomach—crunch-free:

1 BRACE YOUR ABDOMINALS

You have four layers of abdominal muscle, and contracting them when you move—particularly when you're picking up something heavy—will strengthen them and help prevent injury. But contracting your abs is more than pulling in your belly button, McCall says. They should feel as though you're girding to take a punch to the stomach. Imagine trying to tighten a girdle around your middle as you activate all of your core muscles at once.

Over time, this should become a reflex move, so you can brace your abs when you need to without thinking about it, McCall says. This not only strengthens your abdominal muscles, it also protects your back from injury.

2 GET TO THE CORE

McCall recommends adding these core moves to your workout routine.

Bird-dog: Get on your hands and knees with your hands underneath your shoulders and your knees hip-width apart. Raise your right arm and your left leg at the same time until they're parallel to the floor, then reach forward with your hand and backward with your foot. Hold for 2 seconds before returning to the start position. Repeat with the

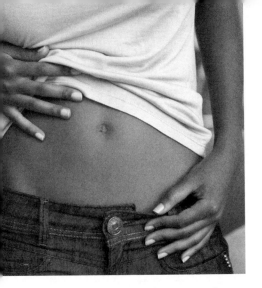

3 GET PLENTY OF CARDIO

"Everybody has 6-pack abs, but some people keep them in a cooler," McCall says. That's where cardio comes in. Brisk walking, jogging, cycling, rope-jumping, cross-country skiing, hiking—anything that gets your heart pumping will burn fat all over your body, including around your middle.

The Centers for Disease Control and Prevention recommend that adults do at least 2½ hours of moderate aerobic activity every week, with strength-training sessions at least twice a week.

4 STOP STRESSING

What does stress have to do with your abs? A lot, as it turns out. Stress triggers the release of cortisol, which causes your body to store fat around your middle. Relieving stress—by getting 7 to 9 hours of sleep a night and practicing relaxation techniques as needed—can help lower cortisol levels and trim your belly. As it happens, exercise is another great way to keep your stress level in check! (For more stress reduction strategies, see chapter 3.)

opposite arm and leg, alternating sides until you've done 8 to 12 repetitions on each side. Work up to two to three sets.

Standard plank: The plank is a fundamental exercise for strengthening and toning your abs because it uses all four layers of muscle between your rib cage and your pelvis, McCall says. Here's how to do it: Begin by lying on your stomach. Brace your abdominals and raise yourself up on your elbows and toes, keeping your body in a straight line from your feet to your head, remembering to breathe. Hold the position 15 to 40 seconds before releasing. Repeat two to five times per workout.

Side plank: Lie on your side with your knees bent and one leg on top of the other. With your elbow directly under your shoulder, contract your abs and push your hip off the ground, keeping your bottom knee on the floor. Hold for 10 to 30 seconds. Repeat two or three times per workout.

Wood chop: For this exercise, you'll need a 5-, 8-, or 10-pound hand weight with which you can complete 8 to 15 repetitions.

Hold the weight in front of you, with your feet shoulder-width apart. Squat down until your thighs are parallel to the floor, making sure that your knees don't go past your toes. The weight should be between your knees. Next, push up through your heels to a standing position, swinging the weight straight up overhead. Do two or three sets of 8 to 15 reps each.

your list ————

—————————————————

—————————————————

—————————————————

—————————————————

—————————————————

—————————————————

—————————————————

—————————————————

—————————————————

—————————————————

5 best moves to tone your arms

mini LIST

Arm stretches

Stretching your muscles will give you a better range of motion and more flexibility. Do these moves after your workout, and hold each one for at least 30 seconds, advises Shaun A. Zetlin, a certified personal trainer.

1. **Triceps stretch.** While standing with your abs tight, raise one arm straight up and bend it at the elbow so that your elbow is pointing toward the ceiling. Tuck your chin, keep your elbow as close to your head as possible, and gently push your elbow closer to your head with your opposite hand. Switch arms.

2. **Wall stretch.** Place your right palm against a wall and keep your left arm at your side. With your elbows locked, pull your body to the left to stretch the right biceps and shoulder. Switch arms.

NEXT TO FLATTENING a bulging belly, tightening flabby arms just may be the most common fitness goal. Let's face it: With trendy sleeveless dresses and camisole tops, "bat wings" are not the most fashionable accessory.

The following routine can help strengthen and sculpt your arms, says Shaun A. Zetlin, a certified personal trainer in the New York metro area. Except for the 21 curls, you'll be doing 2 or 3 sets of 12 to 15 reps of each exercise, with each rep taking about 3 seconds to complete. For those moves that require hand weights, Zetlin recommends using a weight that feels challenging but not over-the-top. In other words, it should be heavy enough that the last two exercises of every set are tough, but you can maintain good form while doing them. If you're cruising to 15 reps without breaking a sweat, then you need to go heavier, Zetlin says.

As with any strength-training exercise, you don't want to work your arm muscles two days in a row, at the risk of overdoing and sustaining an injury. So allow a day of rest before repeating this sequence.

1 WARM UP

Always warm up your muscles first. Simply walk for 5 or 10 minutes on the treadmill or around your house to get ready for your workout, Zetlin says. In order to warm up arms that may have bursitis or an old injury like tennis elbow, Zetlin recommends adding light hand weights to your walk. Hold a 2½-pound dumbbell during your walk in each hand with your arms bent, your elbows tucked in to your sides and gently resting the weights against your shoulders, keeping your wrists straight.

2 TRICEPS KICKBACK

Holding a weight in your right hand, stand with your left foot forward and your left knee bent, making sure that it doesn't extend past your toes. Lean your upper body slightly forward and bend your right arm, holding the weight close to your right armpit. Keep your elbow close to your hip as you slowly straighten your arm behind you, then bring it back to the starting position. Complete the reps with your right arm before switching to your left arm. Work up to 3 sets.

3 ASSISTED TRICEPS PUSH-UP

Changing the placement of your arms in a standard push-up will work your triceps, Zetlin says. For an assisted push-up, kneel on the floor with your knees bent and your ankles crossed behind you, feet up in the air. Lean forward onto your hands, keeping a straight line from your knees to your head and tightening your abs.

Move your arms close to your sides, with your elbows glued to your hips. Lower your body a few inches toward the floor, then return to the starting position. You needn't go all the way to the floor, Zetlin says, but be careful that your hips don't drop and your back doesn't arch.

For more of a challenge, Zetlin recommends doing this move from a standard military push-up position. Lie facedown on the floor with your legs extended behind you. Push up so that you're supporting your weight on your palms and your toes. Keep your abs pulled in and your body aligned from your ankles to your head. Position your arms so that

your elbows are glued to your hips, as above, then lower yourself toward the floor and return to the starting position.

4 TWENTY-ONE CURLS

This move builds the elongated muscle in your biceps, Zetlin says. Stand with your feet hip-width apart and your shoulders pushed back. Hold a weight in each hand, arms at your sides. Pull in your abs, keep your elbows glued to your sides, and curl both hands to belly-button level. Repeat 7 times. Next, keeping your elbows glued to your sides, raise the weights to chest level and lower them only to belly button level. Repeat 7 times. For the final 7 reps, raise the weights all the way to chest level and lower all the way to your sides.

5 PREACHER CURL

In a gym, you would do this exercise using a 90-degree bench that looks like a padded pew at church (hence the name). At home, you can use a soft recliner or a chair with a high back (it should come to about chest level). Stand behind the chair and drape your arms over the back of it, palms facing up, so that it supports your arms, shoulders, and wrists. Tighten your abs and lean slightly forward. With a slight arch in your back and a slight bend in your knees, raise the weights and curl your arms to shoulder level, then lower.

your list

5 butt- and leg-firming moves

mini LIST

Leg stretches

Your workout isn't done until you've stretched. Hold each stretch for 30 seconds, advises Shawn A. Zetlin, a certified personal trainer. If one leg feels tighter than the other, stretch it longer.

1. **Hamstring stretch.** Prop your leg on the back of a sofa or on a chair seat with your toes pointed at the ceiling. Lock your knees, lean forward, and try to touch your toes without rounding your back. Switch sides and repeat.

2. **Quadriceps stretch.** Holding on to a wall with your right hand for support, use your left hand to grab your left ankle and pull your heel to your butt. Switch sides and repeat.

3. **Calf stretch.** Stand on the edge of a step and let one heel drop down over the edge, holding the railing as you do. Switch sides and repeat.

THE EXERCISES PRESENTED here are fantastic for toning your lower body, which also happens to have the largest muscle groups. As for the arm exercises (see page 44), you'll gradually work your way to two or three sets of each move, 12 to 15 reps per set. Each rep should take about 3 seconds to complete.

If you get winded while doing this routine, by all means take a break within or between sets, sitting down if you need to, advises Shaun A. Zetlin, a certified personal trainer. You can continue once you're breathing comfortably again. Remember, too, to give your lower body a day of rest after you do this routine.

1 WARM UP
Begin your workout with 5 to 10 minutes of light aerobic activity, such as walking, Zetlin says.

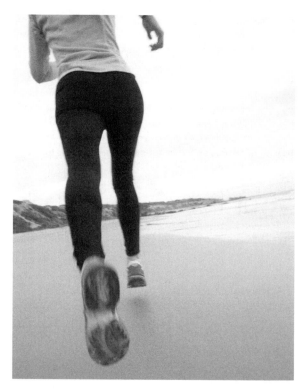

2 STEP-UPS

You can do this exercise on a staircase, holding the railing for balance if you need to. Choose the first, second, or third step, depending how much you want to challenge yourself. The step should be at least ankle-high.

Place one foot on the step and raise yourself up while bringing the other knee forward past your hip. Step back onto the floor, then switch legs. Continue alternating legs for the entire set.

To make this exercise even harder, hold hand weights, cans of soup, or jugs of water at your sides while you step up and down, Zetlin suggests.

3 STATIONARY LUNGES

Stand with your feet shoulder-width apart. Step forward with one leg, holding on to a wall or chair for balance if you need to. Bend your front leg and lower your back knee as close to the ground as possible. Hold for 5 to 10 seconds, then return to the starting position. Make sure that your front knee doesn't go past your toes and that your back heel never touches the ground, Zetlin says. You should be on the toes of your back foot for the duration of the exercise.

4 WALKING SQUATS

Tighten your abdominal muscles and keep a slight arch in your back as you step to the side with your right leg. Squat down until your thighs are parallel to the floor. Your heels should be flat on the floor the entire time. Stand up, bringing your left foot toward your right. Take another step to the right. Continue until you complete an entire set in one direction, then switch legs and work your way to the left.

5 PLANK GLUTE-KICKBACK

Get in the standard plank position by lying on your stomach, drawing in your abs and bringing yourself up on your toes and elbows, keeping your spine in a neutral position. Then bend one knee and bring it as far forward toward your chest as you can without raising your hips or arching your back. Then bring your leg straight out behind you, pointing your foot and raising it a couple of inches toward the ceiling. Hold for one second and go back to the starting position. Alternate legs for one set and rest. Do not do this exercise for longer than 60 seconds without resting, or you could risk hurting your back.

your list

8 tips to stay motivated

my favorite...
Motivator

Kevin McCarthy,
personal trainer

"I've been a runner and a triathlete for 25 years, doing four to eight triathlons and up to 10 runs a year," McCarthy says. "What keeps me going is helping others to reach their goals. I'm active in a running club and triathlon club where I help new runners and triathletes get ready for their first event. And the more social the activity, the bigger the pull for me. I like to get out there and connect with others and build off their energy."

WE ALL KNOW that we should be doing some sort of physical activity most days of the week. Yet when we get caught up in our daily routines, our workouts tend to be the first thing to go to make room for something else. Pretty soon it's been weeks, if not months, since we last broke a sweat—and we're back to square one in terms of slimming down and shaping up.

So much of going out for a brisk walk or heading to the gym is about what's going on inside your head. When your mind isn't in it, sticking with a fitness routine is that much harder.

How do you make your fitness routine stick? Try these strategies for starters.

1 DEFINE YOUR GOAL

Part of what dampens motivation is not having a clear vision of what you want to achieve, observes Kevin McCarthy, a personal trainer, senior health coach, and chief operations officer for First Fitness in Normal, Illinois.

Let's say your motivation for exercising is to lose 25 pounds. You can make it a more defined goal by deciding that you're going to drop two dress sizes in six months, and you're going to do it by taking a spin class three times a week, walking two days a week, lifting weights on alternate days, and cutting calories.

2 FIX AN IMAGE IN YOUR HEAD

If you're exercising for weight loss, you might visualize yourself wearing a smaller size. Are you trying to get back into a pair of jeans that you haven't worn in a few years? Conjure a mental image of yourself slipping in and zipping up, then use it to push yourself to exercise every day, McCarthy says. One of his clients used this technique to slim down for a college reunion. She visualized how she wanted to look when she made her entrance, and that helped keep her on track for her goal.

One caveat with visualization is to be realistic. Don't pine to look like a supermodel if you don't have the genetic material that will get you there. Rather, focus on getting in the best possible shape for your body type.

3 PUT YOURSELF FIRST

Many people don't exercise because they haven't made themselves a priority in their own lives, McCarthy says. We get caught up putting in long hours at work, taking care of family and home, being active in the community, and just being there for everyone else. We have to make up our minds that our physical well-being is worth carving a half-hour to an hour from our daily schedules. If you aren't taking care of yourself, how can you be your best for anyone else?

Some of McCarthy's clients take time every Friday to schedule their workouts for the weekend and the week ahead. "Successful people clear their to-do lists and then start from scratch, writing in what's most important first. Then all the other stuff fills in around it."

4 GET THE GEAR YOU NEED

Take that first step to go out and buy walking shoes and some comfortable workout clothes. Then put everything into place so that you're more likely to follow through with your fitness routine. Rather than trying to pack your gym bag on a busy weekday morning, do it the night before. Set your bag next to your door, or put it in your car. Then when morning comes, it's ready to go when you are.

5 REWARD YOURSELF

Some people are better able to stick with a fitness routine if they give them-selves something to look forward to, says Jessica Matthews, a personal trainer and continuing education coordinator for the American Council on Exercise. For example, you might treat yourself to a manicure or a massage for fitting in your workout every day this week. Matthews recommends setting up weekly and monthly rewards for the first six months of a new fitness routine, while it's still becoming a habit.

6 MAKE EXERCISE AN EVENT

Signing up for a charity 5K or a recreational league sport can be a great motivator, McCarthy says. Let your family and friends know what you're up to, so they can support you.

7 CHECK EXCUSES AT THE DOOR

Don't say that you don't have time to exercise. There are 168 hours in a week, notes Pete McCall, a personal trainer. If you work out for an hour a day, five days a week, that's just 3% of your total hours. Isn't that a modest investment to make in exchange for improving your health and quality of life?

8 HAVE A BLAST

Don't feel that you need to do a certain activity because a certain celebrity is touting it or because everyone else is doing it. "If you hate running, then don't run," McCarthy says. Instead, take a dance class, go mountain biking, or sign up for water aerobics if that's what appeals to you.

When you do what you love, it doesn't feel like work. That may be the most powerful motivator of all. Eventually, you may find yourself craving exercise, not only because it makes you feel better but because you value the "me time" that accompanies a 30- to 60-minute workout. That's when you'll know that you're committed to fitness.

your list

6 strategies to beat workout boredom

my favorite...
Way To Escape the Gym

Michael Wood, certified strength and conditioning specialist, chief fitness officer for Koko FitClub in Rockland, Massachusetts

Wood's tried and true boredom buster is to head outside. He takes his clients for stadium stair runs, hikes, trail running, or jogs on the beach. The key is to scope out your environment for opportunities to exercise in a new way, he says. Head to a sports stadium at a nearby high school or college and start walking the stairs, progressing to jogging and then running. Are there benches at your local park? Do step-ups or push-ups at every third bench. If you live near the beach, run up and walk down sand dunes. You'll increase your fitness and leave boredom in the dust.

DOING THE SAME old fitness routine day after day is no way to get excited about working up a sweat. After all, we already have enough on our plates that's less than stimulating; how about folding laundry or taking out the trash for the umpteenth time? Your workout shouldn't feel like just one more thing that you've got to do.

Changing up your fitness routine not only keeps you from becoming bored, it also gets you in better shape. Over time, your body becomes accustomed to your activity pattern and is more efficient at burning calories while you're doing it, explains Kevin McCarthy, a personal trainer. Now you know why the scale sometimes gets stuck on the same number, even though you're exercising religiously.

There's no reason to trudge through another workout that doesn't inspire you. Whether you have a gym membership or you keep fit at home, there are plenty of ways to mix things up and keep boredom at bay.

1 MAKE IT INTERESTING WITH INTERVALS

When walking or running for 30 minutes has you yawning, try incorporating intervals into your workout. They're easy to do: Just alternate 3 to 5 minutes at a faster pace with 1 minute at a slower pace, McCarthy says. If you're on a treadmill, stationary bike, or elliptical trainer, you can get the same effect by increasing the elevation or resistance for 3 to 5 minutes.

"Your workout will fly by if you think about it in 5-minute intervals," McCarthy says.

2 CHANGE THE TERRAIN

You might be able to inject some vigor into your daily walk by heading for a hiking trail instead of following the same route around your neighborhood, suggests Jessica Matthews, a personal trainer. Or drive to another neighborhood and take in a different view while you work out.

3 CROSS-TRAIN

It's great for getting fit, preventing injury, and eliminating boredom. Rather than slugging through 30 minutes on the treadmill at the gym, stay on for just 5 minutes, then hop on the stationary bike for 5 minutes, then switch to the elliptical trainer for another 5. Go through the entire circuit once more, and you've got your 30-minute workout.

Here's an option for a summertime fitness routine, depending where you live: Jog to the community pool in 15 minutes, swim for 20 minutes, then jog back home for 15 minutes.

4 DISTRACT YOURSELF

In some gyms, you can watch TV while you walk on a treadmill or pedal a stationary bike. Some bikes even have a video display that makes you feel as though you're racing against other people, McCarthy says.

If you have exercise equipment at home, try setting it up in front of the TV to take your mind off of your workout.

5 MAKE EXERCISE A SOCIAL EVENT

McCarthy sees people as fitting one of two fitness personality types: either the loner or the socializer. If you're a socializer, the more people you recruit to work out with you, the better. Join—or even start—a walking or running group. You'll never be bored when you're surrounded by friends.

6 DO SOMETHING COMPLETELY DIFFERENT

McCarthy likes to change his workouts with the seasons. When the weather is appropriate, he switches from running to mountain biking and rock climbing. Here's what you can do:

- **At a gym:** Sign up for classes that you haven't tried before, such as belly dancing, boot camp, or Zumba.

- **At home:** Record a few new routines from TV or invest in a new workout DVD. The American Council for Exercise website (www.acefitness.org) has an entire exercise library online. At Prevention.com, you can download workout videos for your iPod or portable media player.

- **Outdoors:** Expand your fitness horizons by taking wind surfing lessons, visiting a rock climbing gym, going skiing or snowboarding, attending a yoga retreat, or joining an adult dodgeball league. The possibilities are endless!

your list

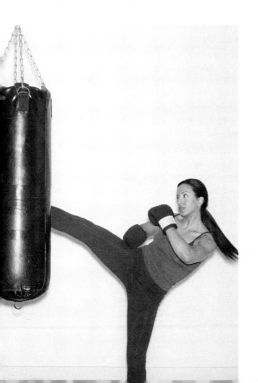

9 tips to find great-fitting shoes

mini LIST

Examine Your Arch

When you're shopping for shoes, take note of the arch of your foot, says Vonda Wright, MD, an orthopedic surgeon.

Before you embark on your shoe search, you may want to examine your footprint by wetting your feet and standing on a piece of paper. If your print looks like:

- **An oval.** You probably have a flat foot with little or no arch, so you need a shoe with lots of support, Wright says.

- **A thin line.** You probably have a high arch, in which the sole of your foot is very curved. You need a more flexible shoe that absorbs shock.

- **Like a footprint out of a magazine.** You probably have a normal foot and can comfortably wear most available shoe styles.

OF ALL OF the fitness gear that you can invest in, your shoes are the most important purchase that you will make. They help to align your entire body, explains Dina Tsentserensky, DPM, a podiatrist and cofounder of NYC FootCare in New York City.

Walking impacts all of your joints: your ankles, knees, hips, back, and shoulders. So when you don't have enough support for your feet, it throws everything else out of whack, Tsentserensky says. Poorly fitting shoes can contribute to blisters, shin splints, knee pain, tendonitis (an inflammation of the tendons that attach muscle to bone), and even stress fractures.

But choosing just the right pair from the several hundred that are available to you—now there's a challenge. These tips can help narrow down your options.

1 SHOP AFTER A WORKOUT

Your feet swell when you exercise, so it's a good idea to go shoe shopping after your workout or after you've been on your feet for a while, says Vonda Wright, MD, an orthopedic surgeon and director of the Performance and Research Initiative for Masters Athletes at the University of Pittsburgh Medical Center. Also, be sure to wear your athletic socks, or buy a pair at the store to try on with the shoes.

2 SKIP THE OUTLETS

To get a properly fitting shoe, you need to go to a store with knowledgeable salespeople who can measure your foot and recommend brands and styles based on your activity, Tsentserensky says. Your best bet is a retailer that specializes in athletic shoes, such as Foot Locker, Sports Authority, or Finish Line. If price is a concern, check out what's on sale.

3 CONSIDER WHAT YOU'RE DOING

Athletic shoes are made for specific activities. The right shoe for your workout will provide good support, enhance your performance, and help protect against injury. If you're engaging in a particular activity for more than a couple of hours a week, Tsentserensky recommends buying a pair of shoes for that activity, whether it's walking, running, tennis, or hiking.

This is especially important if you're running, Wright adds. While you can wear a cross-trainer for walking and most aerobics classes, you should never wear one to run. If your foot isn't well supported when you run, it can change your gait, which can lead to injury, Wright says.

4 GET SIZED
Even if you think you know your shoe size, have your feet measured anyway, Wright says. Your foot changes shape as you age and, if you're a woman, after you have a baby.

5 WIGGLE YOUR TOES
Your athletic shoes will probably be a half-size to a full size larger than your dress shoes, Tsentserensky says. With the shoes on, you should be able to wiggle your toes and have about a thumb's width between your big toe and the toe box.The shoe shouldn't be too tight, but your foot shouldn't slide around in it, either. Because one foot is usually bigger than the other, always buy shoes to fit the larger foot.

6 LEAVE ROOM FOR BUNIONS
If you have a bunion—that is, a bump where you big toe joins your foot—your shoe should be wide enough to accommodate it, Tsentserensky says.

7 CHOOSE WHAT FEELS GOOD
There's no break-in period for athletic shoes, Tsentserensky says. If they don't feel comfortable in the store, they won't once you're exercising, either. If you can, do a bit of your workout while you're in the store. Some retailers have treadmills onsite, so you can try walking or running shoes before you buy.

8 WATCH FOR SIGNS OF IMPROPER FIT
If your shoes give you blisters, it probably means that they're too loose, Tsentserensky says. On the other hand, if your toes feel numb while you're exercising, your shoes may be too small, or the laces may be too tight.

9 REPLACE THEM EVERY 300 TO 500 MILES
By the time you're closing in on mile 300, you'll probably notice that your shoes are starting to lose support, Tsentserensky says. If you don't know how many miles you've put in, judge your shoes by how they feel. Most people can tell if they need a new pair just by the level of cushioning and support their shoes are giving them, Tsentserensky says.

your list

7 steps to find the right sports bra

facts & figures

216
calories

The number of calories burned after playing Frisbee for 1 hour. For comparison, here are the estimated calorie burns for other popular fitness activities, based on someone who weighs 150 pounds:

Running at 10 miles per hour: 1,280

Racquetball: 740

Kickboxing: 720

Singles tennis: 549

Jumping rope: 500

Rollerblading or skating: 477

Soccer: 468

Biking on a flat surface: 441

Walking at 4.5 miles per hour: 440

Hiking: 414

Aerobics: 405

GETTING PROPERLY FITTING shoes is of utmost importance for exercisers. But for women, finding a good-fitting sports bra runs a very close second.

Surveys show that about 60% of women feel breast pain when working out—and in many cases, this may be because of an unsupportive bra. The pure weight of your breasts bouncing up and down can cause back pain, says Vonda Wright, MD, an orthopedic surgeon. And if you participate in a high-impact sport such as running without adequately supporting your breasts, you can permanently stretch the ligaments that attach breast tissue to your chest, Wright adds.

A poorly fitting bra also can cause redness and chafing underneath and on top of your collarbone. You can even get a heat rash underneath your breasts from wearing the wrong bra, Wright says.

So how do you find the right bra for you? Take these tips with you when you go shopping.

1 CHOOSE SUPPORT OVER STYLE

The cute compression-style sports bras may work for young athletes, but older women tend to need more support, Wright says. Follow these guidelines when selecting your bra style.

- If you're an A-cup, a compression bra may work. This bra style—which slips over your head and presses your breasts to your chest—probably provides enough support for smaller breasts.

- If you're a B-, C-, or D-cup, molded cups are best. In this case, a compression bra probably won't give you adequate support, Wright says. Another, even better option: encapsulation bras. They have two separate molded cups, often with extra support from an underwire or a firm chest band. A British study involving 70 women of all cup sizes found that encapsulation bras stopped the breasts from moving in all directions and reduced pain.

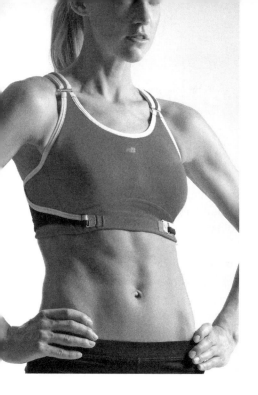

too tight. You should be able to take a deep breath without feeling constricted; otherwise, the bra could compromise your performance when you exercise.

5 CHECK FOR BOUNCE

While you're in the dressing room, take a few small jumps and see what happens. There will always be some bounce, but it should be minimal, Wright says. Keep in mind that a heavier fabric will be more supportive than a lighter fabric.

6 DO A FIT CHECK

If your bra slides up when you raise your arms and touch your hands over your head, it's too tight. If it rides up only in the back, you may need a smaller size.

Make sure that your breasts aren't spilling out of the top or the sides of the bra. With an encapsulation bra, the fabric between the cups should lie flat against your skin. If it doesn't, try a larger cup size.

7 NEED MORE SUPPORT? WEAR TWO BRAS

If you still feel some pain or soreness when you work out, you may get relief from wearing two bras. The best combination: an encapsulation bra with a compression bra over top.

your list ──────

2 LOOK FOR SIGNS OF SUPPORT

Other than the style, certain bra features can help you determine which one is more supportive. For instance, check out the straps; the wider they are, the better. And stretch the fabric. It should have some give horizontally but not vertically.

3 CHOOSE A WICKING FABRIC

A bra that's made from a breathable fabric designed to wick away moisture does make a difference in how comfortable you'll feel when wearing it, especially when you work out in the heat, says Tara Zimliki, a certified personal trainer and owner of Tara's Bootcamp in Branchburg, New Jersey.

4 SLIP IT ON

Once you've chosen bras in a few styles, head for the dressing room to check the fit. The bra should contain your breasts but not smash them, Wright says. The straps shouldn't dig in to your skin, and the overall fit should be neither too loose nor

8 tips for hot-weather workouts

mini LIST

How to recognize heatstroke

Heatstroke is a serious, potentially life-threatening condition. If you spot any of the warning signs in someone, call 911 or seek out emergency medical personnel immediately. While you wait for help to arrive, move the person indoors and have him or her drink cool liquids.

- Body temperature of 104°F or higher
- Rapid heart rate
- Rapid, shallow breathing
- Irritability, confusion
- Skin that feels hot and dry or hot and moist to the touch
- No sweating
- Dizziness, light-headedness
- Headache, nausea
- Fainting (which may be the first sign in an older person)

NO MATTER WHAT the temperature outside, it's going to feel even hotter when you work out. Your body temperature rises as much as 30°F when you exercise, notes Tara Zimliki, a certified personal trainer. So if it's already 80° outside, it may feel like 110° once you get moving.

Working out in hot weather stresses your heart and lungs. Because your body pumps more blood to your skin to try to lower your body temperature, there's less blood for your muscles, so you'll feel more tired.

If it's humid, the sweat on your skin doesn't evaporate as easily, so your body has an even harder time cooling off. You run the risk of developing heatstroke, when your body temperature gets too high.

All good reasons to take the following precautions when the mercury starts to climb:

1 SET YOUR ALARM

In warm weather, move your workout to the wee hours of the morning, Zimliki says. She tries to exercise before 7:30 a.m. in the summer and may head out as early as 4:30 or 5 a.m. on very hot days. Definitely avoid going out for a game of tennis in the middle of the day.

2 SPREAD ON A SPORT SUNSCREEN

Your body has a harder time staying cool when it's sunburned. Use a sunscreen with an SPF of 30 or higher—ideally, one that's waterproof and designed for sports. It will feel lighter, it won't clog your pores, and it won't run into your eyes when you sweat, Zimliki says.

3 CHOOSE YOUR WARDROBE CAREFULLY

Lightweight, light-colored clothes are essential in the heat. Ideally, they should be made from a fabric that wicks away moisture and helps you stay cool in the heat, Zimliki says. Additionally, wearing a visor will protect your face from the sun without making you as hot as a baseball cap would.

4 LOWER YOUR INTENSITY

When it's very hot, skip high-intensity workouts altogether. If you're doing your strength training outdoors, move slowly, Zimliki says.

5 SEEK OUT SHADE

If you can get out of the sun, do it. Find a walking, running, or bike trail lined with trees.

6 TAKE YOUR WORKOUT TO THE POOL

There's no better way to keep your cool while exercising! If you're not accustomed to water workouts, try these for starters:

- **Swim laps.** It's easy to do, and it increases your heart rate for an excellent cardio workout.

- **Run in the pool.** Besides being gentle on your joints, it really gets your heart pumping. Start in the shallow end, where the water is about chest height, and run from one side of the pool to the other. This is a great training activity, and you may notice improvements in your speed and agility once you move your workouts back to land, Zimliki says.

- **Strength-train.** These exercises take advantage of water's natural resistance. First face the side of the pool and hold on. Curl your leg back as though you're kicking yourself in the butt for a hamstring curl, Zimliki says. Do 18 repetitions with each leg. Next, turn around, hold the side of the pool behind you, and lift your leg straight out in front of you for a quadriceps raise. Do 18 repetitions for each leg.

Note that staying hydrated is just as important whether you're exercising in water or on dry land. Keep a water bottle at poolside and take a drink every 15 to 20 minutes.

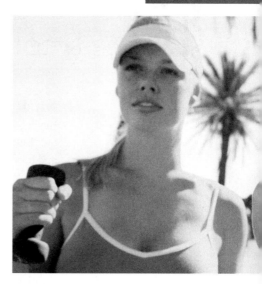

7 STAY INSIDE, BUT TAKE PRECAUTIONS

That basketball game with your buddies can be played indoors instead of out. But gyms get hot and humid, too, which means you should take the same precautions by lowering your exercise intensity and moving more slowly. In the end, your body will be better for it; you'll be stronger than if you worked out hard in the heat, Zimliki says.

8 BRING WATER

Your body needs liquid to produce sweat and cool down. Drink water every 15 to 20 minutes during your workout, Zimliki says. If you're exercising for an hour or longer, drink a sports drink, which will replace the sodium chloride and potassium that are lost in sweat.

your list

10 tips for cold-weather workouts

mini LIST

Power up your workout

Properly fuel your body, and you'll get all of the energy you need for a great workout.

1. **Eat before.** Have a light meal or snack about an hour before you exercise or a bigger meal 3 to 4 hours beforehand. Choose carbohydrates and beneficial fats for energy, and proteins to help repair and build muscle. Good sources of carbs include whole-grain breads, cereals, pastas, rice, starchy vegetables, and fruit. Proteins and fats should come from lean meats, fish, dairy, nuts, and vegetable oils.

2. **Eat after.** A meal consisting of carbohydrates and protein, consumed within 2 hours of finishing your workout, will help repair muscle and replenish your energy stores.

WHEN THE TEMPERATURE drops, you may have the urge to curl up under a blanket and skip your workout. But there are a few advantages to getting dressed and heading outside for exercise.

First, you burn more calories when you work out in the cold, says Tara Zimliki, a certified personal trainer. Your body uses this extra energy to raise your body temperature and heart rate.

Second, it's fun! And getting outside when you're usually cooped up will help brighten your mood during the gloomy winter months.

Third, exercise can help keep you from getting sick during cold and flu season. Research has shown that people who engage in moderate-intensity activity get up to 30% fewer colds than people who don't.

Have we persuaded you to bundle up and head outside? These tips can help winter-proof your workout.

1 GET PUMPED FOR WINTER SPORTS
Cold weather is a great time to try a new, calorie-burning activity. Consider that a 160-pound person can burn 511 calories in an hour of ice skating or cross-country skiing. If downhill skiing is more your speed, it burns 365 calories an hour.

2 CHECK THE OUTSIDE TEMPERATURE
Your body temperature rises by about 30°F when you exercise, so it's okay to work out in cold weather, even for people who have health problems like asthma (though you should get your doctor's OK, just to be safe). That said, once the outside temperature dips below 20°F, especially if there's a windchill factor, you may want to move your workout inside, Zimliki says.

3 DRESS IN LAYERS
Layering is the most effective way to keep warm. Then as your body temperature rises, you can peel off each layer. You'll stay warmer if the first layer is a wicking fabric that pulls sweat away from your skin and keeps you dry. Zimliki recommends making one layer a thermal turtleneck;

that way you can pull the collar over your mouth to warm the air as you breathe.

4 BREAK OUT THE SUNSCREEN

It isn't only for summer. You can get sunburned any time of year, especially if there's snow to reflect the sun's rays. Choose a sport-style sunscreen with an SPF of 30 or higher.

5 COVER UP EXPOSED SKIN

As your body temperature drops, blood rushes to your major organs, leaving your extremities even colder. Stay warm by wearing a hat (up to 40% of heat is lost through your head), along with thermal gloves and socks. Zimliki wears two pairs of gloves in the winter. A headband that covers your ears can also help, she says.

6 WARM UP LONGER

Cold temperatures make for stiff muscles. So if your warm-up usually lasts 5 minutes, extend it to 10 in cold weather, Zimliki says.

7 FOLLOW THE WIND

On a windy day, try to start your walk, run, or bike ride with the wind at your back. Then turn around and head into the wind for the second half of your workout, Zimliki says. By then your body should have warmed up, and you won't be as cold as when you first started out.

8 RAISE YOUR INTENSITY

Cold weather is a perfect opportunity to kick up your workout a notch, because it will help raise your body temperature, Zimliki says. Go for a run instead of a walk, or do higher intensity exercises such as jumping jacks, jump squats (squat and jump straight up), and leap frogs (squat and jump to the side).

9 DRINK UP

You may not feel as thirsty, but you can still become dehydrated from sweating. Sip water even when you don't think you need to. (Experts recommend 2 or 3 cups pre-workout, about 1 cup every 15 minutes while exercising, and another 2 or 3 cups post-workout.)

10 CHECK FOR FROSTBITE AND HYPOTHERMIA

If the skin on your face turns pale or your fingers or toes feel numb or sting, get into a warm building or car as soon as possible. Both of these changes can be early signs of frostbite. Be sure to warm up slowly and refrain from rubbing the area. If the numbness or stinging doesn't go away, seek immediate medical attention.

Likewise, if you're shivering, you have slurred speech, you become very tired, and/or you lose coordination, you could have hypothermia. This also warrants immediate medical attention.

your list

7 ways to get more from walking

mini LIST

Ease into walking

The following steps can help you safely increase the intensity and duration of your walks.

1. **Warm up.** Start with 5 minutes of slow walking.

2. **Then move more briskly.** For your first week of workouts, you'll walk at a brisk pace for 5 minutes. You'll add 3 minutes per workout every week thereafter. So by week 9, you'll be walking at a brisk pace for 30 minutes straight.

3. **Cool down.** End your workout with another 5 minutes of slow walking.

EXERCISE CAN'T GET any simpler than putting one foot in front of the other. Walking is so easy and versatile that you can do it virtually anywhere. All you really need is a good pair of walking shoes.

As with any other type of activity, though, you can get into a rut with walking. Maybe you're not seeing the fitness improvements or feeling the energy boost that you expected.

Try these tips to make your walking workout work for you.

1 CHECK YOUR INTENSITY

Fitness walking is different from everyday walking. You need to push yourself to get your heart pumping; otherwise, it won't do much good.

How do your gauge your pace? Paul McCall, an exercise physiologist, says that you should be moving at a pace at which you can talk but you don't want to. "Having the ability to talk is different from actually talking," he says. If you can't speak clearly, you're pushing yourself too hard. But if you can speak quite easily, you're not working hard enough.

2 STEP UP YOUR SPEED WITH INTERVALS

An easy way to add intervals: Walk as fast as you can for a minute, then slow down for 2 minutes, suggests Shaun A. Zetlin, a certified personal trainer. Repeat this cycle 10 times for a good 30-minute workout. Eventually, you'll be able to maintain the faster pace for your entire walk.

You have a couple of good reasons to pick up your speed. First, it burns more calories. A 30-minute walk at 2 miles per hour burns about 120 calories (for someone who weighs 150 pounds), compared to 220 calories at 4.5 miles per hour.

Second, a faster walk helps melt fat around your middle. A study from the University of Virginia compared women who took three shorter walks at a fast pace and two longer walks at a moderate pace each week to women who walked at a consistent moderate pace five days a week. While both groups burned 400 calories per walk, the women who walked faster lost 2 inches around their waists over the course of 16 weeks. They also lost 8 pounds without dieting—and slimmed down their thighs, too.

3 KEEP TABS ON YOUR STEPS

Counting your steps with a pedometer might be just what you need to fire up your walking workout. Stanford University researchers found that walkers who used pedometers and set a goal of accumulating a certain number of steps took four times more steps and burned 100 more calories than walkers who didn't set a goal. Over the course of a year, that adds up to 12 pounds.

Try wearing a pedometer for three days without making any changes to your walking routine. If you're currently tallying up to 6,000 steps a day (between your walks and other activities), set a goal of 10,000 steps. If you currently rack up more than 6,000 steps, aim for another 5,000.

4 ADD HILLS OR STAIRS

Walking up an incline works your butt, hips, hamstrings, and calves, and it burns more calories, Zetlin says. If you walk outside, map out a route with more hills, or loop around to do the hills more often. If

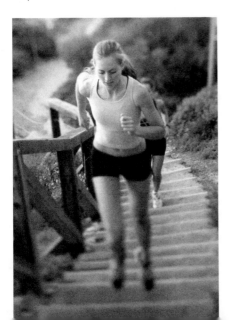

you're a mall walker, taking the stairs can increase your calorie burn.

5 TAKE A HIKE

Simply walking on the uneven terrain of a hiking trail can make your workout more of a challenge and help you use more calories, Zetlin says.

6 WORK YOUR ABS WHILE YOU WALK

Contracting your abdominal muscles and holding them very tight while you breathe through your nose will help you burn more calories during your workout, Zetlin says. He adds that with a strong core, you have more energy, so you can walk longer.

7 HEAD OUT WITH OTHER WALKERS

You'll probably have more resolve to go faster, push harder, or walk longer if someone is willing to do it with you, Zetlin says. Recruit a friend to accompany you on your walks. Ideally, your buddy will be at about the same fitness level as you—though if he or she moves at a faster clip, it may be incentive to increase your own pace.

Another way to find walking partners: Join a walking club. Many gyms offer them. You also can find a group by checking out online message boards on Yahoo and other sites, Zetlin says.

your list

8 questions to ask before joining a gym

facts & figures

33 percent

The amount of improvement in weight-loss results among people who join a gym compared with those who don't.

A GYM ISN'T FOR EVERYONE. But it may be a good option for you if you're looking to diversify your workouts, or you want expert guidance from a personal trainer, or you like to socialize while you work up a sweat.

These days gyms offer the very latest in exercise equipment—such as treadmills and bikes with built-in TVs and video screens—as well as an array of classes from kickboxing to spinning to aerobic dance. Personal trainers are available to teach you proper form and technique. And you'll be surrounded by exercisers who, like you, want to lose weight and get in shape.

The challenge, then, is finding the right gym for you. It pays to shop around, and not just for the cheapest fee or least restrictive contract. The fact is, if you end up not feeling comfortable at the facility you choose, you'll stop going. And that isn't going to help you reach your fitness goals.

Before you sign on the dotted line at any gym, take time to consider these questions.

1 WHERE IS IT?

By far, the most important factor in choosing a gym is location, says Jessica Matthews, a certified personal trainer. "When I talk to people who have fallen out of their fitness routines, I often find that they were enrolled at a gym 45 minutes from their homes," Matthews says. "With all of the things that we have to do on a daily basis, exercise shouldn't be another inconvenience."

2 WHEN IS IT OPEN?

It may seem obvious, but if you plan to exercise in the morning before you go to work, then the gym needs to be open at that hour. Matthews suggests visiting the facility or just driving by at the time of day that you would normally be there. If the parking lot is packed and a line of people is waiting to get on the treadmills, then it may not be the right gym for you.

3 WHAT DO YOU WANT?

Are you looking for classes? Find out which ones a gym offers, and at what times. The classes in which you're interested should be available when you're able to attend, Matthews says.

If you're intending to use the fitness equipment, check out the selection and quality. A gym may have a dozen treadmills, but if only three are functioning, that's a bad sign.

4 DO YOU FEEL COMFORTABLE?

Every gym has a certain atmosphere that can affect how welcome you feel. Some attract a more athletic clientele, which may not be the best place for someone who is just starting an exercise program.

For some women, simply being in a co-ed environment when they exercise is very uncomfortable. If this is the case for you, you may want to look into a women's-only gym, Matthews says. She recalls a client who said that she'd never wear shorts at a co-ed gym, no matter how hot it was. As it turned out, she felt completely at ease wearing shorts and a tank top when she was surrounded by other females.

The staff also will be a factor in your comfort level. When you visit, pay attention to the details, Matthews says. Do the people at the front desk greet you with a smile? Does the staff answer your questions? Is someone available to help you with a piece of equipment?

5 DOES IT HAVE CHILD CARE?

If the hardest part of getting to the gym is finding a babysitter, you may want to look for a facility that offers free child care while you work out.

6 HOW MUCH DOES IT COST?

There's a gym for every budget, from upscale facilities with onsite spas to gyms with more basic amenities—and plenty of price points in between. You should be able to find one that's affordable for you, Matthews says.

7 WHAT ARE THE TERMS OF MEMBERSHIP?

If you're not sure about buying a full membership but you're interested in a few of the classes, ask if you can buy passes just for those sessions.

8 CAN YOU GO ELSEWHERE?

If you just can't find a facility that feels right for you, you do have other options, Matthews says. Many churches, community colleges, and hospitals offer classes to the general public, as do many dance studios.

your list

_____

_____

_____

_____

_____

_____

_____

_____

_____

_____

11 ways to avoid injury

mini LIST

Practice RICE

The go-to remedy for a muscle sprain or strain is RICE:

1. **Rest.** Do this for as long as you're experiencing pain and swelling. If you don't rest the injured area, it may take longer to heal.

2. **Ice.** To reduce inflammation, apply ice to the injury for up to 20 minutes every 2 to 3 hours for 3 days. Be sure to wrap the cold source in a towel before applying to your skin.

3. **Compress.** Control swelling by wrapping the area with an elastic bandage, taking care not to cut off circulation.

4. **Elevate.** Propping the injured area at a level above your heart also helps alleviate swelling.

WHEN YOU'RE MAKING progress on an exercise program, the last thing you want to do is put your workouts on hold because you've hurt yourself.

Always see a doctor if you experience severe pain or numbness, if a joint feels unstable, if a particular body part can't bear weight, or if an old injury begins to hurt or swell. In the meantime, take these steps to stay injury-free.

1 SEE YOUR DOCTOR BEFORE YOU BEGIN

This is especially important if you're age 40 or older; you're overweight; or you haven't exercised for a long time, says Becky Wenner, a certified personal trainer. Your doctor can assess your risk of injury and recommend strategies to protect yourself. You may have forgotten about that elbow injury a couple of years ago, but your doctor will see it in your chart and remind you to avoid overstressing that joint.

2 WEAR THE RIGHT SHOES

Good-fitting, supportive shoes will help you avoid injuries as minor as blisters and as serious as tendonitis.

3 SEEK OUT EXPERT ADVICE

If you're brand-new to exercise, it's probably a good idea to hire a personal trainer or take a fitness class, where the instructor can teach you proper form, Wenner says.

4 WARM UP FIRST

Studies can't seem to agree about whether warming up your muscles helps protect against injury. What it can do is improve your range of motion at your joints and loosen your muscles, so you're less likely to tear them.

Warming up is beneficial in another way: It helps mentally prepare you for what you're doing. That's important, because being distracted and not concentrating on your workout can lead to injury.

5 KNOW THE DIFFERENCE BETWEEN PAIN AND DISCOMFORT

Exercise can be uncomfortable, but the only way to improve your fitness level is to push past the discomfort. On the other hand, exercise should never be painful, and you should never push through pain.

"If you're doing an exercise and you're thinking 'I can't do this' or 'I don't feel like doing this,' then you have to push yourself harder," Wenner says. But if you're experiencing true pain, especially around your joints, you need to stop what you're doing right away. Otherwise, you're putting yourself at great risk for injury.

6 INCREASE INTENSITY SLOWLY

It's been said that you need to walk before you can run, and that's certainly true for exercise. A good rule of thumb is to increase your intensity by about 10% per week.

Let's say that you decide to take up running. You shouldn't lace up your sneakers and head out for a jog if you've never done it before, Wenner says. Instead, start by walking a mile. Then walk 2 miles. Then jog slowly for ½ mile. Once that feels comfortable, you can increase your speed and distance gradually.

7 EXERCISE ALL WEEK, NOT JUST THE WEEKENDS

Weekend warrior syndrome—when you try to squeeze a week's worth of exercise into just two days—is a recipe for injury. It's much better to aim for five days of moderate activity, even if it's broken up into brief, 10-minute workout sessions.

8 LOOK FOR LEVEL GROUND

Walking or jogging on an uneven surface can put you at risk for spraining your ankle.

9 UP CARDIO, STRENGTH, AND FLEXIBILITY

All three are essential to your overall fitness, and to preventing injury. To ensure you spend time on them, develop a schedule that alternates each type of exercise 3 times a week.

10 REST AFTER TRAINING

Your muscles need a day of recovery after you lift weights; otherwise, you could cause a sprain (in which the ligaments that connect your bones at the joints stretch or tear), or a strain (in which the muscle or tendon that connects the muscle to bone stretches or tears), or develop joint pain.

11 KNOW WHEN TO TAKE A DAY OFF

"You're not going to lose your strength and fitness gains just by taking a day off," Wenner says. If you feel that you need to do something, go for a walk instead of running or heading to spin class. When your muscles are tired, they won't support your joints as well, which can lead to injury.

The same rule applies when you're sick. It's okay to work out when you have a runny nose or a cough, but if the illness is below your head—e.g., a chest cold or gastroenteritis—postpone your workouts until you feel better. And, as a courtesy to the other gym members who need to use the equipment after you, be sure to wash your hands frequently and try to avoid touching your mouth and nose and then touching the equipment.

your list ——————

_____

_____

_____

_____

_____

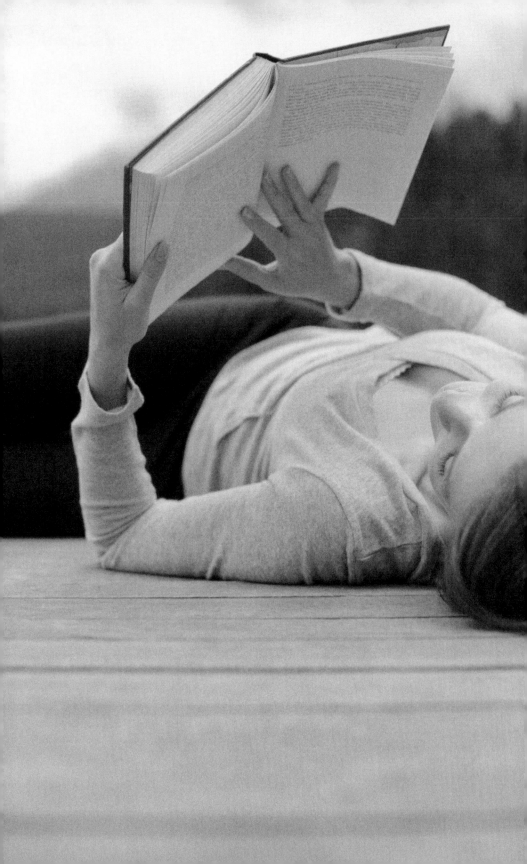

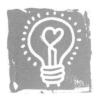

chapter 3 mind

top 10 reasons to stress less

facts & figures

63

percent

The number
of people who believe
their lives are more
stressful now than they
were 5 years ago.

CONTRARY TO POPULAR belief, stress isn't all bad. In modest doses, it motivates us to get things done and keeps us focused on our goals. But when stress persists, as it often does, it can make us physically sick.

"What causes stress may not be the same for everyone," says Bruce S. Rabin, MD, PhD, medical director of the Healthy Lifestyle Program at the University of Pittsburgh Medical Center. He says stressors can vary based on stage of life, socioeconomic level, and marital status, among other factors. Regardless of what's behind your stress, you have good reason—or, perhaps, 10 good reasons—to try to keep it in check. For instance:

1 YOU'LL STAY HEALTHIER

Stress can deplete your immune function, leaving you more vulnerable to everyday ailments like colds and flu, headaches, indigestion, and other gastrointestinal problems. So controlling stress is important not just for your emotional well-being but also for your physical health.

2 YOU'LL LOWER YOUR DISEASE RISK

Persistent, unrelenting stress can weaken your body in such a way that you're more vulnerable to serious chronic illness. For example, stress can aggravate asthma and other lung problems and is a known risk factor for colitis, peptic ulcers, and high blood pressure, which in turn can set the stage for heart disease. "Stress also causes changes in the body that are associated with premature aging," says Melodie R. Schaefer, PsyD, executive director of the Los Angeles campus of The Chicago School of Professional Psychology.

3 YOU'LL EAT BETTER, WEIGH LESS

People under stress tend to not take very good care of themselves. They may slip into poor eating habits just when their bodies most need a little TLC. This is a recipe for weight gain, which can ratchet up stress even more. Stress contributes to overweight in other ways as well, by affecting the body's hormonal and chemical balance. In short, if you're trying to drop a few pounds, keeping a lid on your main stressors is key.

4 YOU'LL EXERCISE MORE

Physical activity stimulates the release of mood-enhancing endorphins, making it the perfect antidote to stress. Schaefer recommends setting a workout schedule. "It adds some structure to your day and reduces your 'stress time' as you focus on other things," she says.
As you begin to notice how good you feel after exercising, sticking with a fitness routine will be that much easier.

5 YOU'LL SLEEP SOUNDLY

A growing body of research is revealing why good sleep habits are so vital to our overall health. "It is during deep sleep that hormones are replenished and cellular regeneration occurs," Schaefer notes. Not surprisingly, stress has a very real—and very negative—impact on our sleep cycle. "It affects the quality and quantity of sleep, which can lead to fatigue," Schaefer says.

6 YOU'LL STRENGTHEN PERSONAL BONDS

In the throes of a stressful situation, you may withdraw from relationships or misdirect your anger and frustration. Your loved ones should be a source of stress relief, not stress, says Amy J. Khan, MD, MPH, medical director for Wellness TotalCare at Concentra, a health-care company in Addison, Texas. Don't hesitate to open up to them about what's troubling you. Your relationship may come out the other side even stronger.

7 YOU'LL BE MORE SOCIAL

When you're under stress, you may not feel like meeting with friends for lunch or a cup of coffee. Before you decline that invitation, though, consider this: Studies have shown that social interactions help alleviate stress. So take advantage of the opportunity to relax and escape your stressor, if only for a brief while.

8 YOU'LL DO YOUR JOB BETTER

At work, unmitigated stress can feed into a vicious circle of unfulfilled promises and unaccomplished goals. "Stress makes it difficult to think clearly, impacting our ability to problem-solve and strategize," Schaefer says. "We may forget about important tasks, make mistakes, and exercise poor judgment." As you learn techniques to harness stress, you'll be able to channel your adrenaline into peak performance in any pressure-cooker situation.

9 YOU'LL GIVE IT YOUR ALL

People who stress are never fully invested in what they're doing. That can lead to even more stress. "It is an endless, very destructive cycle that is solved simply by being in the moment," observes John M. Rowley, director of fitness and wellness at the American Institute of Healthcare & Fitness in Raleigh, North Carolina.

10 YOU'LL BE HAPPY!

Ultimately, controlling stress is at the top of our experts' lists for achieving true satisfaction in life. "Stress can kill our sense of joy and calm, as well as our sense of safety and balance," Schaefer says. Learn how to put stress in its place, and you'll never look back.

your list

7 on-the-spot relaxation techniques

my favorite...
Way to Improve Mindfulness

Diana Winston, director of Mindfulness Education at UCLA's Mindful Awareness Research Center in Los Angeles.

Winston recommends taking a short moment to S.T.O.P.

Stop whatever is happening for a minute, and just press pause.

Take a deep, calming breath.

Observe: What do you notice in this moment? Whether it's an elevated heart rate, tension in your back, or another reaction, simply make a note of it.

Proceed: Now you can continue on where you left off.

FOR WHATEVER REASON—a confrontation with the boss, a fender-bender in the supermarket parking lot, a backed-up toilet just in time for your dinner guests—your emotions sometimes bubble up to the point where they become almost impossible to control. But you can't let these moments get the best of you. The secret to riding the stress wave and coming out relaxed on the other side is a little mind over matter.

The next time you find yourself in an unpredicted pickle, practice one of these expert-endorsed stress-busting techniques. In a matter of seconds, you'll feel calm and in control.

1 FOCUS ON PAST EXPERIENCE

A sunny day at the beach. A cool fall day in New England. Your wedding day. Whatever memory makes you happy and puts you at ease, Michael Ellner, a certified medical hypnotist in New York City, recommends going back there for just a moment. "Imagine yourself soaking up that sense of relaxation and ease, and applying that empowerment to the present situation," Ellner says.

2 MAKE A FIST

No, not to take a swing at someone! In this technique, you let the emotion wash over you before capturing it in your hand, figuratively speaking. "Make a fist with your right hand, tighten it, then release, inhaling and exhaling deeply," Ellner says. "Then vigorously shake those feelings right out of your system."

3 JUST BREATHE

Bruce S. Rabin, MD, PhD, recommends deep breathing as the key to true relaxation. Here's how it's done: Put your right hand on your abdomen and your left hand on your chest, then breathe deeply so that your abdomen rises slightly under your right hand. Take up to 5 deep breaths this way to calm yourself.

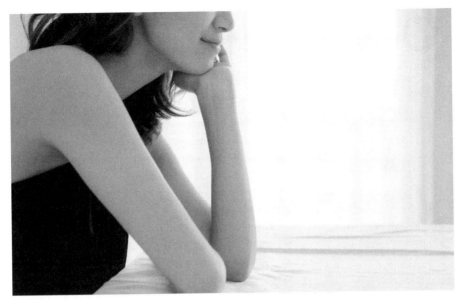

4 TICKLE YOUR FUNNY BONE

Stressors usually aren't funny, but sometimes being able to laugh can defuse a situation. "Select three to five memories that make you laugh, and store them away in your mind," Rabin suggests. "Then when something is upsetting you, go to your 'funny bank' and chuckle to yourself."

5 MAKE LIKE A MONK

Chanting may seem like a strange way to relax, but Rabin swears by it. "The chant can be a religious phrase or just a few words, such as 'I am a good person,' 'All will be well,' or 'I will be well,'" he says.

6 WALK AWAY

The easiest way to calm down and gather yourself in the face of a stressor is to just take a break from it, if only briefly. "Get up from whatever you're doing and walk away," advises B.J. Gallagher, a sociologist and author of *Why Don't I Do the Things I Know Are Good for Me?* "Take deep breaths, shake out your shoulders, roll your head around, stretch your arms and legs, and perhaps go get a cup of tea or coffee"—preferably decaf.

7 GRIN TO BEAR IT

Have you ever seen a football or basketball coach crack a smile at one of the tensest moments of a game? Maybe he or she has heard this advice about how to handle a pressure-packed situation. "Right now, close your eyes and allow yourself to gently smile," says Jennifer Pells, PhD, a psychologist at Structure House Weight Management in Durham, North Carolina. "Your brain will respond by recognizing that you usually smile when you're feeling relaxed and happy. Even if there's nothing in particular to be cheerful about at a given moment, taking a few seconds to consciously smile will send positive signals to your brain."

your list

6 great memory protectors

mini LIST

Stay sharp every day

John Morley, MD, author of *The Science of Staying Young*, notes a number of everyday exercises to maintain a healthy mind.

- Try to memorize any sort of list. At the end of the day, recall as many items as you can.

- Take a sentence from something you are reading and make other sentences using the same words in a different order.

- When you're eating, identify the individual ingredients in your food, including herbs and spices.

- Play video games, particularly ones that require quick responses, with your children or grandchildren.

- Read challenging articles and books, including classic literature and poetry.

- Write a summary of the news you've read or heard that day.

THESE DAYS WHAT'S on many of our minds is, well, our minds. It's understandable, considering the very real risk of Alzheimer's disease (more than 5 million cases in the US alone). But for most of us, an even more realistic risk is the gradual memory loss that tends to occur as we get older—though it can start while we're still in our 20s.

The good news about this type of memory loss is that we can take action to stop it. The secret to preserving memory well into old age goes beyond doing the daily crossword puzzle (although that certainly can help). "The brain responds to novelty, creativity, and invention," says Dorothea Hover-Kramer, EdD, author of *Second Chance at Your Dream: Engaging Your Body's Energy Resources for Optimal Aging, Creativity, and Health*. "Think about the ways in which you can increase your interest in the world around you and ways that you can be of help to others."

For more ways that you can flex your memory muscle, read on.

1 MAINTAIN YOUR SOCIAL CONNECTIONS

One of the best brain-boosting strategies, says sociologist and author B.J. Gallagher, is to keep in close contact with family and friends. "Lively conversations with smart people keep your brain synapses firing on all cylinders," she says. Doing this can be as simple as accepting invitations to family gatherings, scheduling weekly lunches or visits, or calling friends on the phone.

2 LEARN SOMETHING NEW

Several studies have shown that those with less than six years of formal education are at higher risk for developing Alzheimer's disease. While it's unclear whether this is related to the education level itself or to other factors, you can protect yourself by making an effort to expand your intellectual capacity. "At least once a day, challenge yourself to use your brain to remember a phone number, calculate a figure, read a map, or analyze a word for its meaning," advises Jennifer Pells, PhD, a psychologist.

3 MAKE TIME FOR FITNESS

In a recent study of 33 adults ages 55 to 85, those who engaged in aerobic activity four times a week showed improvement in their cognitive function. This is just one of many studies that have linked exercise to cognitive benefit. "A growing body of research is showing us just how important regular physical activity is in terms of protecting our cognitive function as we age," says Pells. Choose activities that are safe and enjoyable for you, and challenge yourself to get better at them.

4 GET YOUR FILL OF FRUITS AND VEGGIES

As for many health concerns, talk of fitness goes hand in hand with another key lifestyle factor: nutrition. "There is not one super-vitamin or mineral that is definitively known to protect your mind and memory because often these nutrients work in conjunction with one another to exert their most beneficial effects," Pells says. "So the best strategy is to focus on increasing intake of the sources of many vitamins and minerals by eating a well-balanced diet. For most people, 'well-balanced' means paying more attention to getting adequate amounts of whole fruits and vegetables"— up to 9 servings, or 4½ cups, each day.

5 PICK YOUR PUZZLE

Crossword puzzles, Sudoku, and similar games are great for exercising your brain, says Bruce S. Rabin, MD, PhD. "Using behaviors to increase development of new connections between brain cells will help to protect memory," Rabin explains. "The behaviors are the continued learning of new things, which may be doing crosswords or Sudoku, or learning to play chess or bridge."

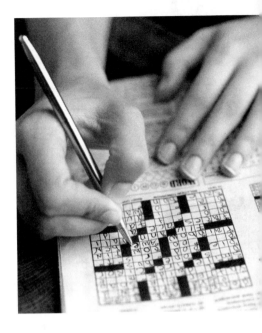

6 BE A MENTOR

One of the best ways to keep your mind fit and your memories fresh is to pass them on to the next generation. "In Africa, the death of an elderly person is considered the death of a thousand books," says Christine Louise Hohlbaum, author of *The Power of Slow: 101 Ways to Save Time in Our 24/7 World*. "So pass on your wisdom. You will benefit, as will your mentee!"

your list

_____

_____

_____

_____

_____

_____

_____

8 clever concentration techniques

my favorite...
Concentration Technique

John M. Rowley, director of fitness and wellness at the American Institute of Healthcare & Fitness in Raleigh, North Carolina

When you need to focus on something, a space with no distractions is essential. But there are other considerations that can enhance or detract from your concentration. Pay attention to your physiology and how you move when you feel that you're on your game. "Some people concentrate best while seated, while others, like me, concentrate best when walking around and engaging their bodies," Rowley says. "Study yourself to see what you do when you are at your sharpest."

MOST OF US have a hard enough time concentrating on the task at hand. Now throw in all of the "conveniences" of modern life–cell phones, text messaging, email, and high-speed Internet—and it becomes next to impossible. Sometimes the distractions are nothing more than annoyance. But they can be a serious concern when they interfere with critical tasks like working and driving.

Thankfully, reclaiming your concentration skills is fairly easily done. You just need to tune in to some things and tune out the rest. Here's what experts recommend.

1 GET ENOUGH SLEEP

That means 7 to 9 hours a night. If you're not sleeping at night, chances are you're not concentrating during the day. "One of the first symptoms of sleep deprivation is poor concentration and diminished cognitive function," says Rallie McAllister, MD, MPH, a family physician in Lexington, Kentucky, and founder and medical director of *The Mommy MD Guides*. "Sleep is critical to maintaining a sharp mind and memory."

2 EAT SMALLER MEALS MORE OFTEN

Our very American habit of eating three squares a day is bad for energy and concentration. It causes our blood sugar to spike after a meal and then take a nosedive in between, giving us a bad case of the mental fuzzies. "Concentration is optimal when the brain has a steady balance of fuel and rest," says Amy J. Khan, MD, MPH. "To improve your performance, consume frequent, small meals rather than eating a few large meals or skipping meals altogether."

3 STAY CALM

If you're angry, upset, or stressed, chances are you're not very focused on the task at hand. Being able to destress is just as important to your concentration as to other aspects of your mental and physical well-being. If you need a few pointers on how to defuse stress effectively, see page 70.

4 BREAK UP BIG TASKS

A large, time-consuming task will tax almost anyone's concentration after a while. That's why Khan recommends dividing it into smaller portions to make it more manageable. "By changing your activity at least once an hour over the course of a prolonged task, you can improve your focus and efficiency," she says.

5 EMBRACE BREAKS

When even divvying up a task doesn't help, get away from it for a few minutes, Khan adds. "Try taking a brisk walk around the office if working on a problem at the computer, or take a short rest if engaged in a precision-focused activity," she says.

6 HAVE A LITTLE COFFEE

"Coffee and caffeine in other forms have been shown to improve concentration and focus, as well as task performance," says B.J. Gallagher, a sociologist. "People do better on tests if they have coffee beforehand. Try chocolate, tea, or cola if coffee isn't your thing." Just keep it to a cup or two, as too much caffeine can have the opposite effect.

7 LET IN THE LIGHT

Do you sometimes feel duller in the winter than you do in the summer? "A simple factor that oftentimes gets overlooked is that the brain is not getting enough exposure to full-spectrum light," says Vaishali, a national health and wellness speaker and author of *Wisdom Rising* and *You Are What You Love*. "There are many high-quality full-spectrum light products available. Improving concentration can be as easy as changing a light bulb."

8 MAKE ASSOCIATIONS

When you can relate a new task to one that you have done in the past, mastering it becomes that much easier, says Thom Lobe, MD, founder and medical director of the Beneveda Medical Group in Beverly Hills. "For example, when you meet someone for the first time, make up a story in your mind that reminds you of the person's name," Lobe suggests. "When you tag new tasks to familiar ones, they are easier to focus on in context."

your list

7 easy ways to think on your feet

mini LIST

Put a stop to performance anxiety

Sharon Jakubecy, a certified instructor in the Alexander Technique, recommends this three-step approach to help you chill out.

- **Expel the air.** Let all of the breath out of your body until you are completely relaxed. "After this, don't suck breath back in," Jakubecy says. "Your body knows how to breathe better than you do."

- **Take a pause.** Next, be calm, quiet, and still for a very brief moment. This needn't be awkward or strange. "The pause gives you the opportunity to calm down," she says.

- **Have a laugh.** Finally, create an internal ice-breaker by smiling and laughing at yourself. "When you laugh at yourself, you can be light-hearted about the situation," Jakubecy says.

PUT SOME PEOPLE in a pressure-packed situation and, just like that, they turn into MacGyver—ready with a plan of action before anyone else gets a chance to say "Now let's think about this for a minute . . ."

Then there are those of us who come up with the snappy comeback the day after the conversation, who stare blankly—like the proverbial deer in the headlights—when we're put on the spot. It's very uncomfortable, even embarrassing. And we'd give anything to be able to think on our feet.

You can sharpen this skill, with the right tools and a bit of practice. Here's what to do.

1 TAKE A DEEP BREATH

If you're in a situation where you feel yourself starting to freeze up, your first step toward regaining control is to pause and take a deep breath, says Amy J. Khan, MD, MPH. "Think about the people whom you care about and who care about you, and at that moment, picture yourself in a comfortable, friendly, nonthreatening place," Khan suggests. "This will give you the composure and presence of mind to make a better choice to respond to the situation."

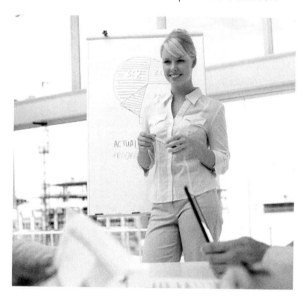

2 REMEMBER: YOU'RE THE EXPERT

When giving a presentation or leading a group, there's probably a pretty good reason for it—and it's because you're incredibly well qualified to be in that situation at that moment. "People tend to forget that they are the experts," says Thom Lobe, MD. "When you need to make a presentation, always remember that you know more about what you are going to say than anyone else. So just have a conversation with your audience, as though you are talking to your spouse, your child, or a close friend."

3 IMAGINE AN EMPTY ROOM

If embracing your expertise doesn't put you at ease, Lobe says many people have success just pretending that no one is there to listen to them. "Mentally block out the audience, and just start talking or carrying out your task," he says.

4 PRACTICE A POWER MOVE

Have you ever seen a basketball player dribble three times before shooting a free throw, or a baseball player go through an elaborate routine before stepping into the batter's box? These are called power moves, and John M. Rowley, director of fitness and wellness at the American Institute of Healthcare & Fitness, recommends using a similar approach to high-stress situations. "Your power move can be something as simple as touching two of your fingers together," he says. "The key is to get yourself into a positive frame of mind and then do these moves over and over again until they are ingrained. Then when you are in a pressure-cooker situation, all you do is touch your two fingers together."

5 PHONE A FRIEND

If you hit a mental block, sometimes the best way to get past is to reach out to someone else, says B.J. Gallagher, a sociologist. "When I have a big project, I always make sure that I have a 'go-to guy' on standby who has agreed in advance to do this for me," she says. "Usually, a 10- to 20-minute conversation will do the trick."

6 GET A GOOD NIGHT'S SLEEP

Nothing can fry your nerves or kill your ability to think quickly quite like being tired, Lobe says. "Get plenty of rest, so you'll be sharp on your feet," he says. "Fatigue tends to exacerbate any form of anxiety."

7 ELIMINATE ANXIETY-PRODUCERS

Lobe also recommends troubleshooting your overall lifestyle to eliminate those things that can cloud your thinking. These include caffeine, excessive alcohol, and cigarettes.

your list ———

———————————

———————————

———————————

———————————

———————————

———————————

———————————

———————————

———————————

8 ways to derail worrying

60 percent

The number of women who worry about paying the bills each month, according to a 2008 Meredith/NBC Universal survey of more than 3,000 women nationwide. Here are some of their other top worries:

Saving enough
for retirement:
75%

Diet and weight:
56%

Credit card debt:
51%

Divorce:
48%

Rising healthcare costs:
46%

WE HUMANS ARE natural worriers. Unfortunately, getting worked up over this or that seldom solves the problem. And it isn't very healthy, either, given the stress and anxiety that it causes.

But we can use worry to our advantage. That's what Kimberly Medlock, a professional organizer, time-management coach, and author of *What Not to Do at the Office: 44 Annoying, Time-wasting and Unproductive Habits in the Workplace*, advises. "Learn how to recognize worry, and then replace it with thinking," she says. "Worry is when your thoughts are stuck on the problem. Thinking is when you are focused on finding a solution. Worry is useless and counterproductive. Thinking is progress and productive."

Of course, we've become so accustomed to worrying that switching off the response takes some effort. These tips can start you on the road to a worry-less existence.

1 DON'T PROCRASTINATE

One way to put an end to worry is to eliminate those responsibilities that lead to worry in the first place. "Many people have a habit of not dealing with issues until they become overwhelming," says John M. Rowley, director of fitness and wellness at the American Institute of Healthcare & Fitness. "Deal with what you have to deal with today. If you are going to procrastinate, procrastinate about worry and procrastination."

2 WORRY PURPOSEFULLY

It's difficult not to think about all that you need to accomplish. So think in a way that leads to results, says Rallie McAllister, MD, MPH. "Decide what you want the outcome to be or what you would like to have happen in the situation that you're worrying about," she advises. "If you don't know what the best-case scenario is, it's difficult to achieve it!"

3 IMAGINE A POSITIVE OUTCOME

Visualize yourself not only dealing with the problem head-on but resolving it successfully, McAllister suggests. "Once you decide what you want to accomplish, visualize it happening," she says. "It takes only a second."

4 GIVE YOURSELF A PEP TALK

Often a little self-encouragement is all that's needed to snap us out of a bout of the worries. "Sometimes we're our own worst enemies," McAllister observes. "You should act as your own coach and best friend, and the voice inside your head should reflect that. Self-talk should always be kind and positive, never critical or mean."

5 SCHEDULE "WORRY TIME"

For some of us, completely eliminating worry is unrealistic. But we can limit it and schedule it, so it doesn't occupy all of our time. Simon A. Rego, PsyD, director of clinical training at the American Institute for Cognitive Therapy in New York, recommends writing down briefly the worry when it occurs. Then, save your notes for a short amount of "worry time" later in the day. "This is a fixed amount of time, such as 20 minutes in the early afternoon or evening, when you intentionally worry about whatever you have jotted down," says Rego.

6 DISTRACT YOURSELF

Another way to override worry is to mentally change the subject. "If you really need to put a stop to worrying, distract yourself," McAllister says. "Engage in an activity that brings you joy or that requires all of your attention."

7 KEEP IT IN PERSPECTIVE

Many of the things that we fret about happen to be things that we have little or no control over. So we need to ask ourselves whether worrying is really worthwhile. "Whatever a constant worrier is worried about, it is likely not as threatening as he or she thinks," says Steven M. Sultanoff, PhD, professor of psychology at Pepperdine University in Malibu, California. "Once a worrier examines the threat and accepts that it is not threatening or that it can be handled, then the worry diminishes."

8 GET REAL

In fact, adds Thom Lobe, MD, a lot of the stuff that triggers worry is almost entirely in our heads. "Often worry relates to personal insecurities that are mostly in the mind of the worrier," he says. "So learn to be realistic. If you can teach yourself to be objective about a situation, you will tend to worry less."

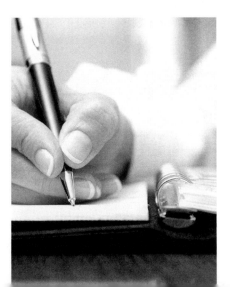

your list ———

_____

_____

_____

_____

_____

7 tricks to bust the blues

facts & figures

18.8
million

Number of American
adults with depression.

80
percent

The number of
people who are not
being treated.

ANYONE WHO HAS ever had depression or has cared for someone with depression knows that it isn't to be taken lightly. Almost 20 million Americans suffer from depressive disorders, and studies suggest that depression will touch everyone at some point in their lives, whether directly or indirectly.

Of course, all of us feel down from time to time. Sometimes the change of seasons triggers it. Researchers estimate that almost 25% of the US population experiences the winter blues, a milder form of seasonal affective disorder (SAD). "Because the hormones involved in SAD and winter blues are closely related to female hormones, women are about three times more likely to be affected than men," says Rallie McAllister, MD, MPH. Other times the stress of work, family, or other lifestyle factors can put us in a funk.

The first step is to make sure you're not suffering from full-blown depression, which is defined as feelings of sadness, loneliness, boredom, irritability or other depressive symptoms that go on all day, every day for two weeks. However, you don't have to wait a full two weeks to see your doctor if you feel like you need help. And if you are experiencing any suicidal thoughts, seek emergency medical help immediately.

For a more ordinary case of the blues, these strategies can help brighten your mood.

1 GET MOVING!

Exercise might be the last thing on your mind when you're down in the dumps, but Margaret Lewin, MD, medical director of Cinergy Health in Aventura, Florida, says there's no better way to snap out of it, whether you go for a brisk walk or spend a few minutes with a Wii Fit. "Physical exercise is the fastest acting antidepressant, raising endorphin levels and allowing the mind to clear," she says.

2 WRITE IT DOWN

Rather than wallow in your emotions, wrap your mind around the feelings and form a plan of action. "Make a list of solutions to what is making you blue, and then make a list of the positive qualities of your life," says Melodie R. Schaefer, PsyD. "Just taking a proactive approach can reduce depression and the sense of hopelessness that sometimes follows."

3 LET THERE BE LIGHT

Particularly during the winder months, lack of sunlight can be a major contributing factor to the blues. "Open curtains and blinds in your home and your office to let in as much sunlight as possible, and turn on overhead lights and lamps," McAllister says. "Sit in a sunbeam whenever you can, and spend more time in the brightest, cheeriest rooms of your home."

4 PICK YOUR PLEASURE

It may seem obvious, but simply doing what you truly enjoy—whether it's woodworking, knitting, gardening, or something else—can get you back to feeling your best. "There appears to be strong evidence that increasing activities of pleasure (things that bring joy to a person) or mastery (things that give a person a sense of accomplishment) can be very helpful," says Simon A. Rego, PsyD.

5 SLEEP, BUT NOT TOO MUCH

In the winter months, it's easy to overdo on sleep, McAllister says. "Many people with the winter blues unintentionally oversleep or sleep in whenever they can get away with it," she notes. "But rising and shining along with the sun each morning increases your daily exposure to bright sunlight, which is incredibly therapeutic."

6 GET SOME GOOD CARBS

Carbohydrates have taken a few knocks in recent years, but they can be beneficial for boosting your mood. The key is to pick the right kinds of carbs. "Although potato chips, chocolate bars, and giant bowls of pasta may be your first and favorite choices, eating too many of these types of foods inevitably leads to weight gain, which can be depressing in any season," McAllister says. "Eating carbohydrate-rich foods is fine, but they should support your health. Good choices are whole fruits and vegetables and whole-grain breads and cereals."

7 TRY A TAG-TEAM APPROACH

Having someone to lean on is always important, but McAllister says that the person should be a full partner in your efforts to defuse the blues. In other words, your relationship should leave both of you feeling better in the long run. "Devise a plan to support each other," she says. "Make regular phone calls and visits to lift each other's spirits, schedule daily walks or exercise sessions, and send each other funny or inspirational e-mails."

your list ———

_____

_____

_____

_____

_____

_____

_____

_____

7 ways to cultivate your inner optimist

facts & figures

89
percent

The number of people who expect the next 5 years to be as good as or better than their current lives, according to a study conducted by the University of Kansas and Gallup. The study involved more than 150,000 adults in 140 countries.

MOODS MAY COME and go, but at the end of the day, some of us are intrinsically "glass half empty" people, while others are "glass half full." And no matter how hard we try, we can't change our tendency to be one or the other. Right?

Margaret Lewin, MD, is one expert who believes that we can. She has seen many a pessimistic person successfully adopt a more optimistic view. She believes that the key is to home in on the qualities that make a person optimistic and try to channel them into your own life.

"Optimists tend to use more problem-focused coping mechanisms, and they're more likely to accept a bad situation and adapt to it," Lewin says. "They also tend to reframe the situation, emphasizing those parts over which they can obtain control, and they often use humor to get past roadblocks."

So now that you know what makes an optimist, how do you go about becoming one yourself? Our experts have offered some strategies that just may fill your glass all the way to the top!

1 ISSUE A HAPPINESS CHALLENGE

Turning yourself from a pessimist into an optimist won't happen overnight. It requires serious and concerted dedication to the effort, much like losing weight or quitting smoking. "Make a list of your thoughts about yourself, your life, and the world," suggests Melodie R. Schaefer, PsyD. "Then challenge yourself to come up with a few thoughts that you would imagine an optimistic person having in the same situation. Start saying them to yourself, and observe how they feel."

2 LEARN TO RECOGNIZE PATTERNS

As you become aware of how an optimistic person acts and reacts, you'll see more clearly how pessimism is manifesting in your own thought processes, says Simon A. Rego, PsyD. Just by being conscious of your thoughts as they occur, you can work on changing them. "Often pessimistic thinking happens so fast that we don't notice it," Rego explains. "It can take a lot of practice to even recognize what we're telling ourselves."

3 FIND THE GOOD IN THE BAD

As you become more conscious of your negativity, you can work on changing it by finding the silver lining in every cloud. "Whenever a new situation or challenge arises, immediately ask yourself, 'What's good about this?'" advises Rallie McAllister, MD, MPH. "If you can't think of anything, or if this exercise feels too awkward at first, try asking yourself, 'What could be good about this situation?'"

4 SURROUND YOURSELF WITH HONEST PEOPLE

Change of this nature is gradual, so it's important to surround yourself with people who are not only supportive but candid. That way, if you do slip up, they'll be sure to let you know about it. "Seeking out people and places that provide us with honest feedback goes a long way toward improving life-long contentedness," says Amy J. Khan, MD, MPH.

5 MEDITATE ON HAPPINESS

In quiet moments, mindful meditation can play a role in changing your outlook on life. "You can repeat phrases that connect with the desire to be happy," says Diana Winston, director of mindfulness education for the Mindful Awareness Research Center at UCLA. "`May I be peaceful and happy,' `May I be at ease'— meditating on these phrases can change the way your brain responds to negative experiences."

6 CONSIDER THE CONSEQUENCES

If all else fails, remember that being a pessimist can be downright devastating to your emotional and physical well-being. According to a study that appeared in the *Journal of the American Heart Association*, women who are pessimistic are more likely to develop heart disease than women who are optimistic.

7 OBSERVE THE POWER OF OPTIMISM

Sometimes being aware of how your optimism can affect those around you is all that's needed to reinforce optimistic behavior. "Words have the power to build up or to tear down, the power to inspire and ignite the spirit or to extinguish a person's internal flame," reminds John M. Rowley, director of fitness and wellness at the American Institute of Healthcare & Fitness. "When you build up the people around you with your words, you also lift up yourself."

your list

_____

_____

_____

_____

_____

_____

_____

_____

_____

_____

_____

7 easy answers for anger

my favorite ...
Way to Rein In Anger

Rallie McAllister, MD, MPH

Sometimes, the people that tend to anger us are doing the very best they can, using the only coping tools and strategies they have. If someone is argumentative or rude, that may be their only way of coping with the present situation. Be the bigger person, and don't fall into the trap of trying to "one-up" the individual. By responding to rudeness with patience and kindness, you may actually teach this person a new way of dealing with difficult situations and have a positive influence on his or her life.

IN THIS POLITICALLY correct world, many of us bottle up our anger, always taking care to put on a cheerful public face. But Steven M. Sultanoff, PhD, reminds us that sometimes a little anger can be a good thing.

"Suppressing anger is considered unhealthy," Sultanoff says. "On the other hand, expressing anger can be useful when it leads to a desired outcome. For example, by expressing anger, you may let someone know that you're dissatisfied with his or her behavior."

Rather than suppressing anger, Sultanoff adds, a healthier strategy is to manage anger, so it doesn't get out of control. That's the goal of the tips presented here. In some cases, though, these may not be enough. If you have trouble reining in your temper, or if it's interfering with your personal relationships, your best bet is to seek professional help, advises Margaret Lewin, MD.

1 MAKE AN EXCUSE

When anger bubbles up, chances are that the next thing to leave your mouth is not going to be good in any way, shape, or form. That's why you need to get out of the situation immediately, says Melodie R. Schaefer, PsyD. "You can tell the person that you will get back to him or her in a few minutes," she says. "Say that you need to make a scheduled phone call, or simply excuse yourself to go to the restroom."

2 TAKE A TIMEOUT

Once you extract yourself from the situation, use the time to collect yourself and calm down. "Try whatever relaxation technique works for you—breathing deeply while counting to 10, repeating to yourself a calming phrase such as 'Take it easy,' or visualizing a relaxing scene," Lewin says.

3 COOL OFF

If a bathroom is close by, a bit of cool water can have an immediate calming effect, Schaefer says. Let it run over

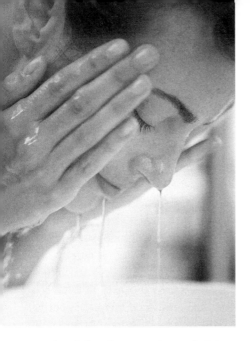

others, lighten the tense mood with a tasteful joke or two. "Just be careful to avoid sarcasm, as that can make things even more toxic," Lewin says.

7 FORGIVE AND FORGET
When dealing with rude people, remember that it isn't about you but rather about whatever is going on in that person's life at the moment. So instead of getting angry in response, show that person some empathy, McAllister says. For example, if a cashier or a bank teller treats you rudely, consider what could be behind her behavior, and put yourself in her shoes. She may have just found out that her husband lost his job, or that her child has gotten sick at daycare.

your hands for a few seconds or splash it on your face. Or head for the water fountain for a nice cool drink.

4 KEEP THINGS IN PERSPECTIVE
When you're seeing red, you may want nothing more than to give someone a piece of your mind, regardless of the reper-cussions. But before you blurt, remember: Is the situation worth losing your job, your marriage, or a friendship over? "Try to put the situation in context," Lewin says. "You don't want to say anything that you'll regret later."

5 CONTROL WHAT YOU CAN
A lot of things that irritate us our beyond our control. So expressing anger about them, while natural, is pretty much futile. "Don't take things personally," says Rallie McAllister, MD, MPH. "If you have car trouble, it doesn't mean that your car—or the world—is out to get you."

6 RELY ON HUMOR
Laughter can defuse almost any situation. So once your nerves have calmed enough to regain control, try to find the humor in what has transpired. If you're with

your list
_____
_____
_____
_____
_____
_____
_____
_____
_____
_____
_____
_____
_____
_____
_____

7 ways to deal with toxic people

my favorite...
Way to Rise Above Toxic People

Melodie R. Schaefer, PsyD

"Don't let yourself get hooked by the bait that a toxic person may dangle in front of you. If someone lays down the gauntlet, you do not have to pick it up. Reacting with hostility and anger or becoming defensive will not help and may cause you to feel you are unsteady in your interpersonal footing. Keeping your balance when dealing with a difficult person can be achieved if you work with your head, not with your heart."

TOXIC PEOPLE ARE like taxes: They're unavoidable. But at least taxes are predictable, coming around at the same time every year. Toxic people . . . well, you never know when you'll cross paths with them. You know the type—the person who is perpetually unhappy and who seems to thrive off the misery of others, including yours.

On this topic, all of our experts agree on at least one thing: Trying to change a toxic person is futile. "When dealing with toxic people, you're better off accepting that they are who they are," says Steven M. Sultanoff, PhD. "It's very important to stay centered and to realize that their toxicity is not in any way going to affect your core value and worth."

Of course, that may be easier said than done, especially when you find yourself face to face with a toxic personality. With these tips, you can survive each encounter with your spirit and self-esteem intact.

1 STICK TO THE FACTS
The best way to deal with toxic people is to keep things as professional, business-like and fact-based as possible—at least on your end. "Stick to the facts of the matter when communicating with the toxic person," says Melodie R. Schaefer, PsyD. "If it seems that they are not able to work toward a resolution with you, suggest taking a break and coming back at a later time to discuss the issue."

2 BRING IN REINFORCEMENTS
If you're trying to work through an issue with a toxic person, sometimes bringing in a third party can turn the tables in your favor. "If you're at an impasse, don't be afraid to consult with someone else," Schaefer says. "If that doesn't work, you may want to have that person present when talking to the toxic person."

3 WATCH YOUR POSTURE
Toxic people will look for the chink in your armor, and that's where they'll attack, trying to chip away at your

defenses. You hold the upper hand as long as you can maintain your composure. "Watch your body language and your posture," says Rallie McAllister, MD, MPH. "Crossing your arms, pounding your fists, and adopting a rigid posture intensify feelings of anger. Take a couple of deep breaths and relax your tense muscles. It will help dissipate mounting anger."

4 FORGET ABOUT REVENGE

It may be fun to imagine getting back at the person who's tormenting you, but retribution is never a good idea. It will ultimately make you look as bad as the toxic person. "Abandon feelings of revenge," McAllister says. "When you focus on trying to get even, you feed into your anger. Let Karma take care of evening the score."

5 HAVE AN EXIT PLAN

If you have time to prepare for the encounter, you can develop a strategy to keep the conversation civil and avoid potential traps, advises Amy J. Khan, MD, MPH. Also, consider how you can end the conversation and exit the situation in case things take a turn for the worse.

6 TURN THE OTHER CHEEK

No matter how much vitriol is being directed at you, let it roll off of you, and turn the tables with a kind word and a smile. Even if it does nothing to change the other person's frame of mind, it will most certainly help yours. "By being kind, you will feel better, and you won't be sucked down by the other person," says John M. Rowley, director of fitness and wellness at the American Institute of Healthcare & Fitness in Raleigh, North Carolina.

7 PRACTICE AVOIDANCE

Of course, there is one easy way to remove all this toxicity from your life and that's to stay away from the person creating it. "Life is too short to surround yourself with toxic people, which is why my number one advice in this area is to avoid the person if at all possible," says McAllister. The only problem is that this is not always possible. "If it's a friend, family member, or coworker, don't be afraid to seek out counseling or advice from others in the office, including your boss, if the situation becomes unbearable."

your list

_____

_____

_____

_____

_____

_____

_____

6 solutions to life's biggest stressors

mini LIST

Less stress in 1-2-3

No matter what is behind the stress in your life, Jennifer Pells, PhD, has a three-step approach that can help.

1. **Assess your stress.** Make a list of all your stressors. Then rate them on a scale of 1 to 10 according to how much each one bothers you.

2. **Get to the source.** Spend some time reflecting. "Once you have a clearer sense of what is stressing you the most about a given situation, you can begin to take specific steps to address it," Pells says.

3. **Build in buffers.** These help protect against your daily stressors. Schedule fun or relaxation for yourself, or pass stressors to others who can help.

NO MATTER HOW many relaxation techniques we have in our personal arsenals, sometimes they're no match for the big-ticket stressors that we encounter. According to a recent survey by the nonprofit group Mental Health America, personal finances are the most common source of stress, followed closely by health and work.

The trouble with major stressors like these is that we never get a break from them. In the long run, they can set the stage for even more problems, especially as far as our health is concerned. "Reacting to life circumstances with a stress response can occur spontaneously with such frequency that we don't realize we're experiencing stress until it causes physical symptoms, such as headaches, high blood pressure, and gastrointestinal problems," says Melodie R. Schaefer, PsyD.

This is why it's so important to stop these stressors from getting the best of you. Consider what's driving most of the stress in your life, then devise a plan of action to keep it in check. These tips will get you started.

1 FINANCES: LOOK AT THE BRIGHT SIDE

You may not see any good in being strapped for cash. But it's all a matter of perspective. "To me, one of the more positive aspects of our current economic situation is that it's bringing families closer together," says Rallie McAllister, MD, MPH. "When we're trying to pinch pennies, we're more likely to stay at home and spend time with our loved ones. It helps us to rediscover what's really important."

2 WORK: STAY AHEAD OF THE CURVE

Employees often know when a big layoff is just around the corner. In this situation, the best strategy is to plan ahead, says Margaret Lewin, MD. "Do the best you can to retain your current job while actively seeking a fallback," she says. "Think about negotiating a severance package. Do a skills inventory, and update your resume.

Keep an eye and ear open for personal and professional contacts."

3 WORK: EXPLORE NEW OPPORTUNITIES

If you get a pink slip despite your best efforts, don't sink into despair. After all, it may be a blessing in disguise. "When my friend lost her job, she was devastated and afraid, but she decided to start her own business. Within a few months, she matched her old salary, and within a few years, she more than doubled it," McAllister says. "Crisis forces us to make changes, and in most cases, they can be for the better."

4 HEALTH: LEARN, THEN TAKE ACTION

Serious health problems, whether our own or a loved one's, can send us into a downward spiral of despair. According to McAllister, the best way to take control of a health crisis is with education and action. "Learn all that you can about the condition that is stressing you," she says. "If your child is diagnosed with diabetes, educate yourself about it. Once you have a good understanding of it, you are aware of your options and can make the best decisions."

5 FAMILY: DON'T GO IT ALONE

When family crises occur, we have an unfortunate habit of shutting out the people around us and trying to shoulder the burden ourselves. But Lewin believes that there is no better time to bring the family together, so you can each help each other. "If a loved one passes away, don't try to cope alone," she says. "Recruit others to help you organize and prioritize a list of needs. Then delegate as much as you can, using your energies to supervise your helpers."

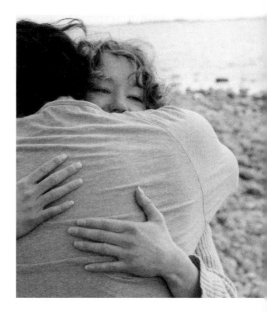

6 GLOBAL CONCERNS: DON'T LOSE ANY SLEEP

Many of us list the economy, wars and politics among our biggest stressors. But in this case, it may be time for a reality check. "Global worries should be categorized into those totally beyond your control—and then pushed out of your mind entirely—and those toward which you can contribute," says Lewin. Contributing can be as simple as giving money or time to your favorite charity, recycling more, or voting in a local election.

your list

9 amazing confidence builders

my favorite . . .
Fact about Failure

Steven M. Sultanoff, PhD

"Failure and confidence may seem mutually exclusive, but the reality is that confident people don't hide from failure," Sultanoff says. "In fact, they embrace it! People who are self-confident are confident in their success and equally confident in their failure because they accept their failures as part of life's experiences. So accept that it's okay if you fail. It may not be what you want, but if you don't succeed, you are still valuable and worthy."

HOW WE RESPOND to stress often boils down to how we feel about ourselves. People with high self-esteem are able to bounce back from problems more easily. But for those with low self-esteem, bad news can make them feel even worse about themselves.

The curious thing about low self-esteem is that people who have it may not realize it. "Our thoughts tend to form patterns and become such potent reflexes that we are not even aware of what we are saying to ourselves about ourselves," says Melodie R. Schaefer, PsyD.

The key to breaking this cycle of self-doubt is to adopt an entirely new mind set, one that boosts our confidence and reinforces our ability to deal with the crisis at hand. "We need to challenge the thinking that eroded our confidence to begin with," Schaefer adds. Here's how.

1 COMMIT TO GROWTH
Learning, doing, achieving—all of these things help you to grow as a person and, as a result, increase your self-confidence. "Expand your horizons by taking part in new activities that use your considerable skills, challenge you to develop new ones, and expand your social network," says Margaret Lewin, MD.

2 FOCUS ON YOU
As vain as it may sound, when you look good and feel good, you will have more confidence. To that end, Lewin recommends taking a lesson on applying makeup, getting advice on your wardrobe, or hiring a personal trainer.

3 LEARN TO IGNORE "THE VOICE"
To gain confidence, you need hit the "mute" button on that negative voice inside your mind. "It may not even be yours!" says Rallie McAllister, MD, MPH. "It may be the critical voice of a teacher, a coach, or a parent. Listen to it one last time and decide if it's your voice or someone else's. Then refuse to listen to it again and drown it out with a positive thought or idea."

4 SAY SOMETHING POSITIVE

"Make a list of at least 30 positive statements about yourself," Schaefer suggests. "Then keep the list in a place where you can see it and read it to yourself or out loud. Notice how you feel when you read it, and how you feel over time as you continue to engage in this practice of positive self-affirmation."

5 PAMPER YOURSELF

You work hard, so taking a break to reward yourself will further reinforce your self-confidence. "Buy a special treat for yourself. It can be something small, like a scented bar of soap or a favorite tea," Schaefer says. "When you use the soap or drink the tea, take a moment to celebrate your gift and to acknowledge the person you are."

6 WRITE DOWN YOUR TO-DOS

McAllister recommends making a list of your daily tasks and crossing off each one as you go. "A visual reminder of all that you've accomplished is incredibly empowering," she says.

7 DON'T COMPARE YOURSELF TO OTHERS

Your self-worth should not be based on how you measure up against someone else. "All of us have distinct personalities, skills, and circumstances," McAllister says. "We can follow different paths and timelines to the same destination."

8 DO GOOD THINGS

Donate to the Red Cross. Volunteer in a soup kitchen. Such experiences add to your self-worth. "People who do good things feel good about themselves," says B.J. Gallagher, a sociologist.

9 RADIATE SUCCESS

"When you are confident, you move more deliberately, speak a little surer, breathe a little deeper, walk a little quicker. You may even have a bounce in your step," says John M. Rowley, director of fitness and wellness at the American Institute of Healthcare & Fitness. "If you are not feeling quite so confident, start moving, talking, and breathing like you are. Before you know it, you will be!"

your list

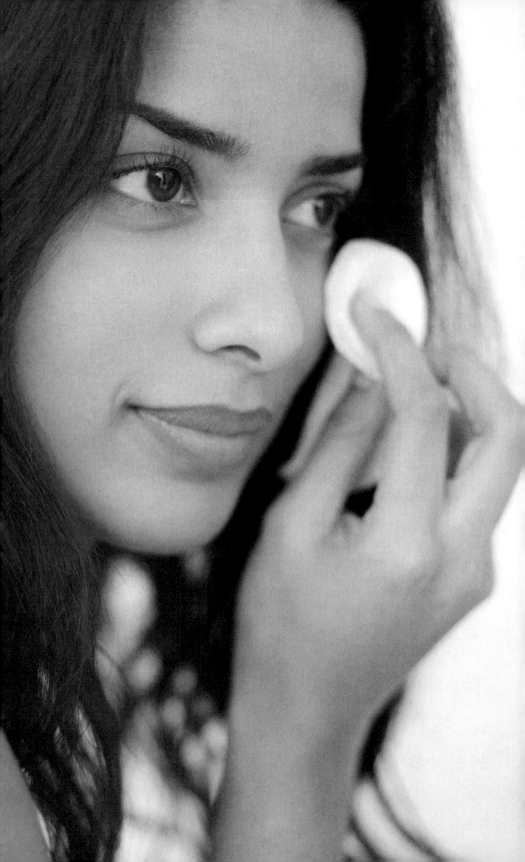

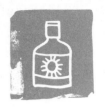

chapter 4 beauty

top 10 steps to look your best

my favorite ...
Skin-Care Gadget

Elizabeth K. Hale, MD, a board-certified dermatologist and clinical associate professor of dermatology at New York University School of Medicine

A good facial cleansing at bedtime is very important, Hale says. "Personally, I use Clarisonic, an electric skin cleansing brush. It has revolutionized my skin-care routine." Clarisonic is designed to remove dirt and oil, soften and smooth skin, and minimize pores and wrinkles. "I used to think that my face was clean at night, but now that I've been using this product, the difference in my skin is unbelievable," Hale says.

THE AVERAGE AGE at which women become proactive about their appearance: 50. But it is never too early—or too late—to put your best face forward. After all, when you like what you see in the mirror, it shows in how you present yourself to rest of the world. To let your natural beauty shine, no matter what your age, use these tips as your foundation.

1 LIVE BEAUTIFULLY

"Remember that beauty comes from the inside as well as the outside," says Francesca Fusco, MD, a board-certified dermatologist in private practice in New York City. "For a more healthful glow, do all of the things your mother told you to do—get enough sleep, avoid cigarettes, de-stress with meditation and exercise, drink plenty of water, and eat a balanced diet."

2 MOISTURIZE FROM THE INSIDE

Without sufficient oil, your skin becomes very dry and tired-looking. "Postmenopausal women, in particular, need essential fatty acids in their diets," says Richard A. Baxter, MD, a board-certified plastic surgeon in Seattle. Omega-3s—from foods such as oily fish (such as salmon), walnuts, and raw almonds—are an integral component of the membranes that surround your skin cells. They help to restore suppleness and heal rough, dry skin.

3 MAKE AN APPOINTMENT FOR PAMPERING

Fusco recommends seeing a dermatologist annually for consultation and treatment. "A microdermabrasion or chemical peel as little as once a year can really make a difference," she says. "Plus, you can get insider information about the newest and latest things that you can do to improve your skin."

4 PLUCK WITH CARE

Carefully groomed brows can make your face look brighter than unkempt ones. "But if you over-pluck your brows, the hair may not grow back," says Ramy, a New York City–based makeup artist and brow artist. That's why he suggests a professional brow shaping. "Having it done by an expert offers you the objectivity that you don't have when looking at your own face. Then you can maintain your brows at home until you feel you need a touch-up."

5 INVEST IN THE ESSENTIALS

Neal Schultz, MD, a board-certified dermatologist based in New York City, identifies three must-have products for healthy, radiant skin: a gentle chemical (glycolic) exfoliant, an antioxidant cream, lotion or serum, and a sunscreen. "The antioxidant and sunscreen protect your skin from the sun's damaging rays, while the combination of exfoliant and antioxidant will leave your skin smoother and more lustrous," Schultz says.

6 BECOME A CREATURE OF HABIT

"Regardless of which products you use, following the same skin-care routine twice a day, every day, will significantly improve your skin tone and texture and reduce acne breakouts," Schultz says. The only difference between your a.m. and p.m. rituals should be the type of moisturizer you use; Schultz recommends using a moisturizer that contains a sunscreen with an SPF of 15 to 30 in the morning, and a product that contains an antioxidant at night.

7 TREAT YOUR HAIR WITH HOT OIL

From the sun's damaging rays in the summer to indoor heat and static electricity in the winter, every season takes a toll on your hair. "That's why I believe regular hot oil treatments are so important," says hairstylist Paul Labrecque, owner of Paul Labrecque spas in New York City. "They help your hair retain moisture while keeping the cuticle closed." You can get a hot oil treatment at a salon or spa, or ask your stylist to recommend a product for home use.

8 ERASE A FEW YEARS INSTANTLY

"If you are getting ready for an evening out, grab your thickest, richest moisturizer, put some in a microwave-safe dish, pop it in the microwave, and heat it up for about 10 seconds," Fusco says. "Then apply it like a mask and let it sit on your face for about 5 minutes before wiping it off. Your skin will be all plumped up."

9 USE THE BARE MINIMUM

If you are in a hurry and want to look fresh in an instant, Hollywood makeup artist Scott Barnes recommends touching up with eye drops, mascara, an eyelash curler, and lip gloss.

10 GO GREEN AND GLOW

If you have a history of allergic reactions to some skin-care products, or if you simply prefer to use only natural substances on your skin, look for the organic designation on product labels. Organic products contain fewer of the ingredients known to cause reactions. Find these top organics at your local pharmacy or department store:

- Juice Organics Vitamin Antioxidant Serum
- Kiss My Face Big Kiss Organic Palm Oil Soap
- Pangea Organics Facial Mask
- Origins Organics Nourishing Face Lotion

your list

7 ways to prevent sun-damaged skin

my favorite...
Sun Protection

Elizabeth K. Hale, MD, a board-certified dermatologist

Sunscreen is a wonderful invention, but it isn't a substitute for physical barriers to the sun's harmful rays. "For ultimate protection, you should wear a hat and sunglasses and stay in the shade whenever possible," advises Hale. "I personally love the sun and swimming, but I never go outside without a hat and sunglasses. I even wear a hat when I swim in the ocean."

IN A WAY, we don't have any more control over the sun's effects on our skin than we do over whether the sun will shine on a given day. "When it comes to protecting their skin from the sun, I tell clients to select their parents. After all, genetics plays a huge role in determining what type of skin we have and how it is subject to damage," says Howard Rosenberg, MD, a board-certified plastic surgeon and skin health expert in Mountain View, California.

You can't choose your parents, obviously. But you can get an upper hand on your genes by making sure to safeguard your skin against the sun's harmful rays.

"Year-round sun protection is important," agrees Elizabeth K. Hale, MD, a board-certified dermatologist. Most everyone packs sunscreen for the beach. But scientists now know that even on a cloudy winter day, up to 80% of the sun's ultraviolet A (UVA) radiation can penetrate through the clouds, reflect off of the snow, and reach your skin through a window. "UVA radiation contributes not just to skin cancer but also to skin damage, photo-aging, and hyperpigmentation—all of the undesirable things that people come to see me to get rid of," Hale says.

Here's how to shield your skin all year round.

1 APPLY SUNSCREEN EVERY DAY

Look for a broad-spectrum sunscreen—meaning that it blocks both UVA and UVB rays—with an SPF of at least 30 (or higher in the summer months) and apply it to all sun-exposed areas, Hale says. If you want to kill two birds with one stone, wear a moisturizer that contains sunscreen. And don't skimp. "Studies have shown that people don't use enough sunscreen for an SPF 30 product to be effective," Hale says. "You need a really good coating of about 2 milligrams of sunscreen per square centimeter of skin, which is a lot."

2 TREAT YOUR HANDS LIKE YOUR FACE

Unless you wear gloves, your hands are exposed to the sun's rays every single day. "Skin cancer is common on the backs of the hands, as are sunspots. Every day women come into my office and ask me to remove brown spots from the backs of their hands," Hale says. "But both skin cancer and spots can be prevented by coating your hands with sunscreen every day."

3 SHIELD AGAINST UVA AND B WITH C

"Vitamin C is an antioxidant. Although it doesn't act as a sunscreen per se, it does help neutralize the deleterious effects of UV rays on your DNA," says Francesca Fusco, MD, a board-certified dermatologist. More precisely, vitamin C works by neutralizing the free radicals that contribute to wrinkling, brown spots, and other skin changes. In one study, women who applied vitamin C cream to their sun-damaged skin for six months saw less discoloration and fewer fine lines. So when you get up in the morning, Fusco says, wash your face, put on a vitamin C serum, and apply a sunscreen over that. Then you're ready to face the day's rays.

4 TOUCH UP WITH MAKEUP

Certain mineral makeup powders have sunscreen built right in. "It isn't always practical to take off your makeup and add another layer of sunscreen," Fusco observes. "With an SPF mineral makeup powder, you can brush on a little added protection throughout the day."

5 WATCH FOR SOD

"Superoxide dismutase (SOD) is a chemical that buffers the effect of UV rays and reduces redness and sun damage,"

Fusco explains. "It is new and just starting to appear in some creams. It's an exciting development."

6 PAINT YOUR NAILS

According to the Skin Cancer Foundation, sun can damage the nail bed and even cause skin cancer under the nail. Wearing a colored nail polish can help block the sun's rays. "For the best coverage, look for a polish with UV filters built in," Hale says.

7 DON'T IGNORE YOUR DOME

The top of your head gets the most direct exposure to the sun, so you should take extra precautions to protect it. To prevent sunburn, the best thing you can do is wear a hat. If you prefer not to, the next best protection measure you can take is to massage sunscreen directly into your scalp. "Choose an oil-free sunscreen to avoid greasy hair," Hale says. In the winter, you can safeguard your scalp and preserve heat, too, by wearing a warm hat.

your list

6 tips to erase wrinkles

mini LIST

Rx wrinkle treatments

If you don't mind making an investment, a multitude of wrinkle treatments are available through your dermatologist. Here are three from Howard Rosenberg, MD.

1. **Chemical peel:** Causes skin cells to regenerate. Chemical peels range from daily treatments that do a little more than exfoliate to phenol peels, which completely remove the outer layer of skin (wrinkles and all).

2. **Dermabrasion:** Uses a diamond-encrusted sander to literally sand down the skin. Most often used to remove fine lines around the lips.

3. **Intense pulse light treatment:** Uses light to treat sun-damaged skin.

FOR SOME OF us, wrinkles are visible reminders of past transgressions—perhaps too many hours in the sun without sunscreen, or too many cigarettes. For others, they reflect a lifetime of emotions—smiling, frowning, and furrowing our brows. Whatever their cause, wrinkles are not welcome. They make us look, and feel, old before our time.

"Obviously, the best thing that you can do for wrinkles is prevent them in the first place," says Elizabeth K. Hale, MD, a board-certified dermatologist. Above all else, that means using a broad-spectrum sunscreen (SPF 30 or higher) every day without fail, and wearing a hat and sunglasses whenever practical.

But even if the skin damage is already done, we have some control over how early those lines appear and how deeply they settle in. With some input from our experts, we've put together this list of proven wrinkle-fighting methods:

1 GIVE SKIN AN A

"Topical vitamin A products, called retinoids, have been shown scientifically to build up elastic fibers and collagen under the skin and reduce wrinkles," says Howard Rosenberg, MD, a board-certified plastic surgeon. Retinoid products are available by prescription—Retin-A is one example—or over the counter. Good OTC products include Neutrogena Dermatologica Retinol NX Serum, RoC Multi-Correxion Night Treatment, and Olay Professional Pro-X Deep Wrinkle Treatment (which is better for sensitive skin). "If you've got wrinkles and you want to use skin-care products to treat them, retinoids are your best bet," Rosenberg says.

2 SEAL IN MOISTURE

Always apply your moisturizer while your face is damp. "Your skin is like a sponge," explains Francesca Fusco, MD, a board-certified dermatologist. "If you put moisturizer on a dry sponge, it will be a dry sponge with grease on it. But if you soak the sponge in water, the sponge plumps up and the moisturizer seals in that plumpness."

Your skin is most hydrated right after you get out of the shower, so that is your best time to moisturize. If for some reason that isn't possible, then wet your fingers under the faucet, pat your face, and put on your moisturizer.

3 RELAX

When you're under stress, it shows up on your face immediately in the form of a furrowed brow and squinting eyes. These subconscious expressions can leave behind permanent lines. "Plus, skin is inherently healthier without circulating stress hormones," says Richard A. Baxter, MD, a board-certified plastic surgeon.

You can buffer your entire body against the physical effects of stress by following a healthy lifestyle that includes getting 7 to 9 hours of sleep every night, avoiding excess alcohol and caffeine, and eating a diet rich in fruits, vegetables, and whole grains. For more stress-busting strategies, see page 70.

4 CURB YOUR SWEET TOOTH

Not only do sugary foods put on the pounds, turns out they can also make your skin look dull and wrinkled. During a natural process called glycation, sugars in your blood attach to proteins and form substances called advanced glycation end products (AGEs). These AGEs damage the collagen and elastin in your skin, which help keep skin firm and youthful. So next time you're tempted by a candy bar, doughnut, or other sweet, bolster your willpower by envisioning young, healthy skin.

5 PERK UP WITH PEPTIDES

"Peptide-containing creams and serums stimulate collagen production," says Neal Schultz, MD, a board-certified dermatologist. More collagen equals smoother and firmer skin. One such product is Olay Regenerist Daily Regenerating Serum.

6 REVITALIZE WITH VITAMIN C

"Vitamin C serum really works to fight wrinkles," Rosenberg says. It not only neutralizes the free radicals that can lead to sagging, wrinkling, and other skin changes, it also helps fade brown spots and smooth and firm skin. Look for a serum product that lists vitamin C near the middle of the ingredients list or higher; this means that the product contains the minimum 5% concentration of the vitamin necessary to produce benefits.

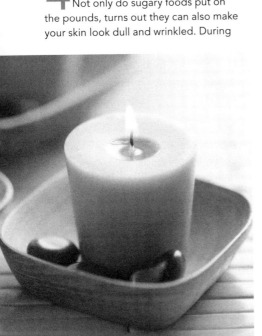

your list
_____
_____
_____
_____
_____
_____
_____

8 clues to determine your skin type

facts & figures

Up to

90

percent

The number of women who think that they have sensitive skin. "In reality, most of these women probably have sensitivities to ingredients in certain products and are self-inducing their sensitive skin," says Elizabeth K. Hale, MD, a board-certified dermatologist.

THERE ARE TWO main categories of skin typing: one that assesses the risk of skin cancer, and another that indicates the skin's tendency to be oily, dry, combination, sensitive, or acne-prone.

"In terms of skin cancer, the Fitzpatrick skin type scale rates how much melanin pigment you have on a scale of I to VI and, therefore, how likely you are to burn," says Elizabeth K. Hale, MD, a board-certified dermatologist. Someone with very light skin and eyes, who always burns and never tans, gets a rating of I. At the other end of the spectrum is someone with dark skin that never burns and only tans; this person gets a rating of VI. The higher the rating, the lower the skin cancer risk—though Hale emphasizes that no skin type is completely exempt from cancer.

The other, more familiar skin typing isn't nearly so cut and dried. "Skin type is influenced by age, menopause, and even the season, so a single strategy may not always be useful," says Richard A. Baxter, MD, a board-certified plastic surgeon. "Not all skin-care analysis is rocket science, though. Women generally know if they have oily or dry skin."

Because many skin-care products are tailored to certain skin types, knowing which type you are can affect how you cleanse and moisturize. Heed this advice before heading for the cosmetics counter or beauty aisle.

1 INSPECT FOR OIL

"Pretty much anyone can recognize if he or she has oily skin," says Francesca Fusco, MD, a board-certified dermatologist. "If you wake up to greasy skin or notice oil on your face after being up for only a few hours, you are an oily skin type."

2 PERUSE FOR PIMPLES

"If you have had pimples, black-heads, whiteheads, or undersurface bumps on your face in the past 3 months, or if your skin tends to be extra-oily, you have acne-prone skin," says Neal Schultz, MD, a board-certified dermatologist.

3 SCAN FOR SIGNS OF DRYNESS

Take a good luck at your skin in a mirror in the middle of the day. "If the skin on your cheeks—but not next to your nose or between your eyebrows—is dry, flaky, or tight, you have dry skin," Schultz says.

4 SEE BOTH SIDES OF YOUR SKIN

If you've experienced pimples in the past 3 months, and you see occasional signs of dryness, such as tightness or flakes, chances are you have combination skin, Schultz says.

5 NEITHER OILY NOR DRY?

Accept being normal. After all, it's a blessing. "People with normal skin are neither prone to acne breakouts nor overly dry—an indication that facial oils are in balance," Schultz says.

6 ASSESS FOR SENSITIVITY

"If different skin-care products frequently irritate your skin, causing redness, swelling, or even pain, you probably have sensitive skin," Schultz says. People with true sensitive skin can have a hard time finding products that they can tolerate. If you experience only an occasional reaction, however, you may have sensitivity to certain products but not sensitive skin in the true sense of the term.

7 FACTOR IN YOUR AGE

As you get older, your skin may take on characteristics of all of the types. But it is most likely to become extra dry. "If you are 'of a certain age' and the skin on your entire face—including the T-zone of your forehead, nose, and chin—is dry, flaky, or scaly and very difficult to keep hydrated, then you have what is called mature skin," Schultz says.

8 WHEN IN DOUBT, SEE A PROFESSIONAL

If you're still not sure of your skin type, evaluation by a dermatologist is probably the way to go, Baxter says. "For example, at my clinic, we use a digital multi-spectrum analysis called VISIA that measures skin type and several different manifestations of aging. This allows for selection of treatments and products on a scientific basis," he says.

your list

7 essential skin-care products

my favorite . . .
Skin-Care Strategy

Francesca Fusco, MD,
a board-certified
dermatologist

"Every woman should
use a topical exfoliant at
least once a week to
slough off dead skin
cells," Fusco says.
"It can be a physical
exfoliant, which has little
granules in it, or a
chemical exfoliant in the
form of a peel that you
apply at home." Start
out exfoliating once a
week. If you can do it
more often without your
skin looking red, raw, or
rutty, go ahead. But as
soon as you notice
irritation, cut back.

YOU CAN'T TURN on the TV or flip through a magazine without seeing an ad for the latest breakthrough skin-care product. From de-puffing under-eye rollers to anti-acne systems to $700 wrinkle creams, there certainly is no shortage of options to pamper and perfect your skin. Perhaps the biggest challenge is deciding how best to spend your beauty dollars. On your behalf, we asked our experts: Which products should no one be without? Here are their top picks.

1 SUNSCREEN

"No one should ever leave the house without applying sunscreen, even if it is raining or snowing," says Elizabeth K. Hale, MD, a board-certified dermatologist. "It should be part of your regular routine, like brushing your teeth." She recommends wearing an oil-free product like Coppertone Oil Free Faces SPF 30 under your foundation or tinted moisturizer (which, ideally, should also contain sunscreen).

2 MOISTURIZER

For daytime, use a moisturizer that contains ceramides as well as sunscreen, advises Francesca Fusco, MD, a board-certified dermatologist. "Ceramides are an indication that the product has really good moisturizing properties," she says. If you want anti-aging effects as well, choose a moisturizer with either antioxidants or peptides. "You also should look for a moisturizer labeled as non-comedogenic, so it won't clog your pores," Fusco says. For best results, apply your facial moisturizer right after you get out of the shower to lock in moisture.

3 RETINOIDS

Retinoids are vitamin A derivatives that boost collagen production and speed up cell renewal, thus preventing dull, blotchy skin. "Apply a few drops of a retinol product at night, after you wash your face. Then follow with a nighttime moisturizer," Hale suggests. "If your skin can tolerate prescription-strength, try something like Retin-A. Otherwise, use an over-the-counter product

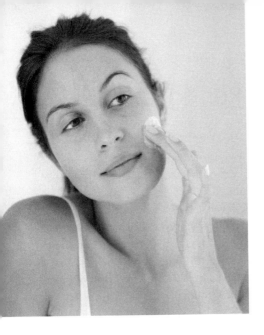

expensive and inexpensive lip balms don't differ much from one another, so this is one place that you can save some money," Fusco adds.

7 HYDROCORTISONE CREAM
Every woman should keep some over-the-counter 0.5% hydrocortisone cream in her medicine cabinet, Fusco says. "If you have any redness, or even a big fat red pimple, applying hydrocortisone cream will reduce the inflammation in a pinch," she says. "You can't use it every day, but it works nicely in an emergency."

your list

containing the ingredient retinol. OTC products are less irritating." Hale adds that a number of companies make good OTC retinol products, including RoC, Oil of Olay, and Estee Lauder.

4 PORE CLEANING STRIPS
If you don't have the time or the budget for regular facials, Fusco suggests the pore cleaning strips sold in drugstores as an effective alternative. "Used once a week, they very nicely extract blackheads from the forehead, nose, and chin of all skin types," she says.

5 EYE CREAM
If you have sensitive skin, you should purchase a separate moisturizer for around your eyes, Fusco says. "The skin around the eyes is very thin, and creams are made with special ingredients that won't cause any irritation," she explains.

6 LIP BALM
"A quality lip balm that keeps lips nicely moisturized is essential," Fusco says. You may opt for the kind that contains petrolatum, usually sold in drugstores, or one of the more expensive waxy balms available in department stores. "But really,

9 skin-care mistakes to avoid

my favorite
OTC Skin-Care Products

Elizabeth K. Hale, MD, a board-cert professor of dermatology

Don't let your skin-care regimen break your budget. "There are a handful of very good expensive products available, but for the most part, I believe in products that you can buy at your local drugstore," Hale says. You can get a good sunscreen, retinoid product, and moisturizer—all for a decent price.

Bear in mind, too, that many major cosmetics companies have more expensive product lines under their corporate umbrellas. For example, L'oreal owns Estée Lauder, Lancôme, and other brands, and some of the Lancôme products are very similar to what you can get over the counter under the brand name L'oreal. You just have to be a smart shopper to find them.

AS MUCH AS we want to trust that all of the skin-care products sold in drugstores and department stores live up to their claims, the fact is, certain ones should be avoided—either because they're not safe or they're not suited to your unique skin type. As you evaluate your current skin-care regimen, remember: The purpose of skin care is to protect the skin barrier, says licensed esthetician Lydia Sarfati, CEO and president of Repêchage and skin-care council director of Intercoiffure salons. "Be gentle with your skin and use ingredients that hydrate, nourish, balance, and rebuild," she advises. And steer clear of these skin-care don'ts.

1 DON'T MIX SKIN-CARE APPLES AND ORANGES

"Avoid putting any products meant for your body on your face," says Francesca Fusco, MD, a board-certified dermatologist. Products designed for use on the body contain ingredients that could potentially irritate more delicate facial skin.

2 DON'T BORROW

"Avoid using skin-care products that have been prescribed for someone else," Fusco says. These products require prescriptions for a reason, and they could be harmful if used by someone for whom they weren't intended.

3 DON'T USE PRODUCTS WITH LONG INGREDIENTS LISTS

Generally, products that contain fewer but better quality ingredients are best for your skin. Also, "if you have a reaction to a product with a long ingredient list, you won't know which ingredient was the culprit," says Richard A. Baxter, MD, a board-certified plastic surgeon.

4 DON'T USE TOOTHPASTE ANYWHERE BUT YOUR MOUTH

A popular home remedy is to apply toothpaste to a pimple to make it heal faster. "Actually, it can burn your skin," Fusco says.

5 DON'T DOUBLE UP ON EXFOLIANTS

"If you use a granular exfoliant, apply it with your fingers or a washcloth, not with a buff puff or something that has its own exfoliating properties," Fusco says. Too much sloughing will irritate your skin.

6 GET A DOC'S OK TO TRY HYDROQUINONE

Hydroquinone is a common ingredient in products for hyperpigmentation, the medical term for brown spots. Previously available only by prescription, it is now available over-the-counter as well.

"When used under the guidance of a dermatologist, hydroquinone can be a very beneficial topical agent for removing skin discoloration," says Elizabeth K. Hale, MD, a board-certified dermatologist. "However, there is a subset of women who will develop deposits of pigment in their skin in reaction to hydroquinone—the exact opposite of the effect they were going for," Hale says. So if you want to try a product made with hydroquinone, be sure to do so only with medical supervision.

7 DON'T OVERDO ANTI-AGING

Layering too many anti-aging products on top of each other can be counterproductive, Fusco cautions. "For instance, don't use an alpha hydroxy acid wash followed by a glycolic acid pad followed by a retinol product—you will irritate your face," she says.

8 DON'T FALL FOR THE QUICK FIX

"Watch out for instant plumpers," says Neal Schultz, MD, a board-certified dermatologist. "They may make wrinkles look better for a few hours, but each time you use them, they cause the skin to swell (that's how they make lines and wrinkles 'magically' disappear). This repeated swelling and shrinking stretches elastic fibers, eventually causing skin to sag and become even more wrinkled."

9 DON'T WASTE MONEY ON COLLAGEN

"Any product that contains collagen or elastin is a complete waste of money. The collagen doesn't get incorporated into the structure of your skin," Baxter says.

your list

7 steps to choose your perfect foundation

my favorite...
Foundation Ingredient

Elizabeth K. Hale, MD, a board-certified dermatologist

"I personally recommend foundations with sunscreen. Because they contain SPF, they provide a bonus layer of protection for your skin." Ideally, your face is getting enough SPF from your sunscreen or moisturizer. But if not, your foundation can make up for the shortfall. "You simply can't have too much sun protection," Hale adds.

SOME WOMEN USE foundation to brighten their faces and even their skin tone, while others rely on it to hide major imperfections. And there is a product for every purpose. The challenge is finding the best one for your skin and your skin-care concerns. These tips take some of their guesswork out of finding the right foundation for your face.

1 DETERMINE YOUR COVERAGE
"For light coverage, look for a tinted moisturizer or makeup labeled as 'sheer,'" says Neal Schultz, MD, a board-certified dermatologist. If you want heavier coverage, a cream foundation is your best bet.

2 FIND YOUR TYPE
"It is very important to choose a foundation that correctly matches your skin type," says Schultz. His advice:

- If you have oily skin or are prone to breakouts, look for an oil-free, matte, or powder foundation.
- If you have dry skin, choose a foundation that contains moisturizer. Also, go half a shade lighter, because oils from your foundation will mix with your skin and make it look darker.

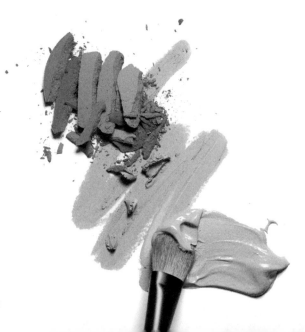

- If you have combination skin, go with an oil-free foundation that contains moisturizer.

3 CHECK THE SHADE

Some women try to match foundation to the color of the skin on the backs of their hands or the insides of their wrists. A better place to test a product, though, is along your jaw line, says Francesca Fusco, MD, a board-certified dermatologist. Your neck is where the makeup will blend in to your normal coloring, so by matching the shade to the skin in this area, you will get the most natural, even look. "Make sure that the foundation blends in well," Fusco adds. "You shouldn't see a dramatic difference between your jaw line and your neck."

4 TAKE IT OUTSIDE

"To best match color, I advise people to go to a window and look at themselves in sunlight—not indoors, with all the funky lighting," Fusco says.

5 NOTE YOUR TONE

It's important to choose a foundation that suits both your skin color and your skin tone. They're two different things. "Most product lines offer colors for fair/ivory, medium/beige, and bronze/dark," explains Schultz. "Within these broad groups are several tones, which are meant to help balance your skin and create a more neutral palate. The difference has to do with undertones, such as yellow, orange, and pink. In most cases, the yellow-toned foundations will provide the most natural look."

6 DON'T BREAK THE BANK

"Do you get what you pay for when it comes to foundations? Absolutely not," Fusco says. There are major companies like Loreal that own sub-companies like Estée Lauder and Lancôme, whose foundations are much more expensive. "And a lot of these products are very, very similar," she says. Savvy women know that some of the Lancôme foundations are similar to what you can get in a pharmacy for a lot less money—you just have to be a smart shopper to find them, she says.

7 KEEP YOUR BEAUTY ROUTINE BACTERIA-FREE

"I am not a fan of foundations that come in compacts and collect bacteria to be reapplied to the skin," says licensed esthetician Lydia Sarfati. "Instead, apply foundation from a bottle with a disposable foam applicator, not with your fingers. Touching the liquid in the bottle will contaminate the remaining foundation, and touching your face with your fingers introduces bacteria to your skin."

your list

_____

_____

_____

_____

_____

_____

_____

_____

_____

_____

_____

_____

_____

10 tips to find a good stylist

mini LIST

Red flags to watch for

If you notice any of the following during your initial consultation with a stylist, don't hesitate to walk away:

- Lateness
- Lack of confidence or knowledge
- Gum chewing
- Gossiping
- Pushiness
- An unclean or otherwise unkempt appearance
- Distractedness
- An inability to listen or communicate well
- A lack of education
- An obvious push to sell the latest trend or product

YOUR HAIRSTYLIST IS much more than the person who does your hair. When you spend hours sitting in his or her chair, the two of you develop a rapport. Over time, your stylist may become a confidant and a friend. Accordingly, says Naz Kupelian, a Boston-based salon owner and platform artist for the RUSK creative design team, the most important attribute to consider when choosing a hairstylist is good communication skills.

"For the stylist, it is not just about the haircut or color, but about building a relationship and being really honest with the client," Kupelian explains. "Ultimately, you don't want a stylist who will readily copy the haircut from a picture that you brought with you if it won't flatter you. You want a stylist who will tailor a cut and color to you and create something that will help you look your best."

What else can you do to be sure that you're putting your hair in the right hands?

1 SCOPE OUT STYLES

If you see someone with a hairstyle that you love, ask for the name of his or her stylist, says hairstylist Paul Labrecque. Then contact the salon where the stylist works and request a consultation. "A good stylist will always allow you to come in for a consultation," Labrecque says. "This is such an important step, because although the stylist did well by the person whose hairstyle you admired, your hair could be nothing like that person's."

2 TAKE YOUR SEARCH ONLINE

"Go on the web and search for hair salons in your area," suggests Anthea Metzger, vice president of Full Circle Studio, a cut and color salon in Cleveland. "You will get more information and photos than you'll find in the phone book." Then, once you've identified a few salons that you like the looks of, call and ask for a little background on their stylists.

3 PERUSE THE REVIEWS

"While you're online, take time to read any comments that customers have posted," Kupelian says. "It is really important to find a salon about which the clients are happy enough to write positive reviews."

4 REMEMBER: OPPOSITES ATTRACT

This is especially true when it comes to choosing a stylist. "If you have a very strong opinion of how your hair should look, you need to find someone who respects that opinion," says Labrecque. "If you don't have a strong opinion, you want a stylist who will lead the way and tell you what will and will not look good on you."

5 MAKE SURE YOUR STYLIST KNOWS WHEN TO STOP

"Try to find someone who you know wouldn't do something to compromise the integrity of your hair," Labrecque says. "Once your hair has been damaged, you can do conditioning treatments to make it look better temporarily, but it won't really come back for at least 2 years."

6 ESTABLISH A MAINTENANCE SCHEDULE

"A good stylist will help you understand the care required for your cut and color, so you have a general idea of how often you should go back for maintenance," says James Corbett, owner of the James Corbett Studio & Spa in New York City. For example, he or she should clearly indicate the maximum number of weeks that you can go between color treatments, highlights, and cuts.

7 ASK FOR AT-HOME ADVICE

"Your stylist should assess your hair and provide guidance on how you can maintain your style yourself," Corbett says. "For example, an air-dry, wash-and-wear style will look completely different when smoothed, styled, and blown out. Your stylist should understand that and help you recognize your home styling limitations."

8 HOLD OUT FOR PATIENCE

"This should go without saying, but find a stylist who is patient and not rushed," Corbett says. "He or she should take time to listen to and understand your needs."

9 LET YOUR STYLIST KNOW THE WHOLE YOU

When creating your hairstyle, a good stylist will account for not only your coloring and facial shape but also your career and fashion sense, Corbett says.

10 DON'T BE AFRAID TO CHEAT

On your stylist, that is. "If you're going to a salon that you like but you aren't happy with the stylist that you chose, don't hesitate to look around the place for someone else that you could try," Metzger says. "After all, salons are about customer service."

your list ———

—————————————
—————————————
—————————————
—————————————
—————————————
—————————————
—————————————

8 must-have hair-care products

my favorite...
Hairbrush

Paul Labrecque, owner of Paul Labrecque spas

"Everybody should have a boar bristle brush, because boar bristles polish the cuticle and help spread sebaceous oils. So as you are drying and shaping your hair, you are also making it healthier." Boar bristle brushes are available in most salons and online. Check the label to make sure that the brush is made with 100% boar bristles.

WITH ALL THAT we have on our plates, we still manage to spend an awful lot of time and energy on our hair. Some of us don't mind spending an hour in front of the mirror with a round brush and dryer; others simply want to wash and go. Either way, we care a great deal—probably more than we'd like to admit—about how our locks look. And when our hair doesn't cooperate, it can quickly send the day into a downward spiral.

Persuading our hair to do what it should on a consistent basis begins with the right products, properly used. Here's what our experts recommend.

1 LISTEN TO YOUR STYLIST

"Some clients spend a lot of money on their color and cut but then use cheap hair-care products. It doesn't make sense," says salon owner Naz Kupelian. Ideally, you should use products especially for your hair type (i.e., oily, dry, color-treated, fine). The only way to do that, Kupelian says, is to follow your stylist's product recommendations.

2 PROTECT YOUR COLOR

"A good shampoo for color-treated hair will help maintain your color for the 8 or so weeks between appointments," Kupelian says. You may spend a little more money on the product, but you end up saving because you'll be able to stretch out the time between colorings.

3 PLUMP UP YOUR HAIR

If your hair is on the fine side, a quality thickening product will give it more volume, Kupelian says. "Apply it before you blow dry," he suggests.

4 POLISH IT, TOO

To really boost shine, Kupelian recommends a pure silicone product. Silicone coats and smoothes the cuticle, so hair reflects light evenly and appear shinier. If you have thick hair, try a silicone serum; if your hair is fine, go for a silicone spray.

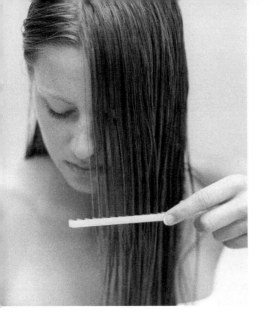

5 BUY IONIC

"Ionic hair dryers (and other styling tools) put less heat on your hair, so they cause less damage than regular hair dryers," says hairstylist Paul Labrecque. Appliances that use ionic technology are made with tourmaline, a type of stone that generates negative ions, which reduces styling time and, therefore, heat exposure. "Ionic dryers still blow warm air, but the very front of the dryer doesn't get hot," Labrecque explains. "So if you press the hair dryer against your hair, you won't get a burn or a singe."

6 GO GREEN

If you care about the environment as much as you care about your hair, you may want to look into the "green" styling tools now on the market. "For example, Rusk has come out with Go Green flat irons and blow dryers made from recycled plastic and decorated with soy ink," Kupelian says. "They also have features that use 30 to 40% less energy." The flat iron, for example, automatically cools from 450°F to 130°F if it's left on for a while without being moving. Hot Tools and Vidal Sassoon are two additional companies that offer energy-efficient styling tools.

7 SEAL BEFORE YOU STRAIGHTEN

Flat irons damage your hair, period. If you absolutely must use one, first add a protective layer in the form of a straightening gel or balm. "Our Straight Style straightening gel (www.paullabrecque.com) contains plant mucilage, which is the inside of the stamen of a plant," Labrecque explains. "It leaves a very fine film on the hair that when heated, creates a protective layer between the hair shaft and the iron." Another good product is Protective Oil by GHD (www.ghdhair.com). "You spray it on your hair to add protection," Labrecque says.

8 MOISTURIZE WHILE YOU SHAMPOO AND CONDITION

"Even people with oily roots tend to have dry ends," Labrecque says. "And when you have dry ends, you need to put some moisture back into your hair." An easy way to do that is with a moisturizing shampoo and conditioner. Labrecque suggests looking for products that list water as one of the first ingredients, "because you want to put water back into your hair." Also, look for panthenol or B vitamins, which will seal the cuticle and hold in moisture.

your list ─────────
────────────────
────────────────
────────────────
────────────────
────────────────
────────────────

7 hair-care products to avoid

facts & figures

53 percent

The number of women who say they spend more time trying to control frizzy hair than they do exercising.

IN ORDER TO keep our hair looking good, we treat it pretty badly—blow-drying, highlighting, perming, and straightening so that it does things it wouldn't do naturally. Unless we're careful, all that abuse can become counterproductive, causing serious damage that takes weeks or months to undo.

For the sake of your mane, be wary of these hair-care products and tools.

1 NYLON BRISTLE BRUSHES

"They're not good for your hair. They conduct heat, and they don't spread oils," says hairstylist Paul Labrecque. Instead, he recommends a brush made with 100% boar bristles to polish the hair's cuticles and spread sebaceous oils.

2 FLAT IRONS

These apply heat directly to the hair shaft, which burns and dries out the ends. "My advice is to avoid flat irons altogether—but if you absolutely must use one, choose a model like GHD's (www.ghdhair.com)," Labrecque says. "It has a computer chip that reads the thickness of your hair and adjusts itself to the appropriate heat level." Also, apply a straightening gel or balm before styling your hair, and never flat-iron more than twice a week.

You can get a flat-iron look without the damage with a new treatment available in some salons called the keratin permanent blow dry. "It makes your hair dry so that it looks as though it was ironed," Labrecque says. The treatment washes away in 3 to 4 months. It costs between $350 and $700, depending on the length and thickness of your hair.

3 CHEMICAL TREATMENTS

"Chemicals are your hair's enemy," Labrecque says. "Too much bleach, color, or relaxer causes a lot of damage." As a rule of thumb, you should allow 7 to 10 weeks between chemical treatments, at bare minimum. And when you do go in for a touch-up, make sure that your stylist treats only the regrowth rather than pulling the processed hair through once again, Labrecque advises.

4 HOME COLORING KITS

"Most over-the-counter hair colors are meant for use on hair that's 100 percent gray," says salon owner Naz Kupelian. So if you apply a medium brown color to hair that is only 50% gray, the parts that aren't gray will come out black. "You may save $50 to $100 in the short run, but in the long run, you will spend $300 to $400 to fix the color professionally," Kupelian says.

Also, don't become a color chameleon. "When you find a color that you like, stay with it," Labrecque says. "When a client is constantly changing her color—a little lighter this month, a little darker next month—it forces the stylist to continuously overlap color to the ends, which causes a lot of damage."

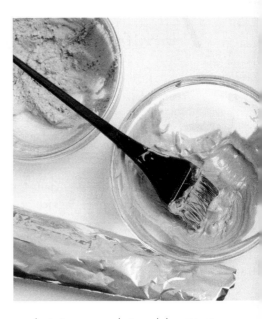

5 PERMS

Labrecque says he seldom sees clients getting perms anymore. That's a good thing, because keeping permed hair healthy is a challenge. "When hair is wrapped in a roller, the hair that has been permed before can't be separated from the hair that hasn't been permed before," Labrecque says. What's more, a person with shoulder-length hair will get three to four perms over the course of 2 years to maintain her style. By then the ends will look terrible.

6 WAX

"Although it may make your hair look better in the short term, wax tends to build up over time, eventually causing your hair to become brittle," Labrecque says. "The same goes for products that contain alcohol."

7 BARGAIN BRANDS

This is one product category where price can be a reflection of quality. "If you see a cheap price, it's a cheap product," Kupelian says. You can buy salon-quality products in supermarkets and drugstores, but if they're the real thing, they'll cost the same as in a salon. "So you may as well buy them where your stylist can suggest the best products for you," Kupelian says.

your list

7 tips to get a good manicure

mini LIST

5 signs of a bad nail salon

These days you can find a nail salon on just about every corner, so you can afford to be choosy when deciding where to schedule your appointment. A poorly run salon can put you at risk for fungal infection, among other health and safety concerns. If you notice any of the following, Green Celebrity Nail Stylist Jenna Hipp says, they're your cue to pack up and go elsewhere.

- The smell of harsh fumes (the salon could be poorly ventilated, forcing you to breathe in dangerous chemicals)

- A manicure or pedicure that hurts or feels invasive

- A technician who cuts your cuticles

- Tools that appear to not have been properly cleaned or disinfected

- Pedicure tubs that are reused without being scrubbed and disinfected first

FOR WHAT AMOUNTS to a little polishing, buffing, and moisturizing, a manicure certainly can deliver a lot of mileage, especially in terms of making a good first impression. "I always say that you can tell a woman's age by her hands, so taking care of your hands and nails is very important," says Suzi Weiss-Fischmann, vice president and artistic director of OPI. "Luckily, nail polish is one accessory that is always in and always affordable."

To polish your nails and, thus, your overall appearance, you can get a professional manicure or do your own at home. For her part, Weiss-Fischmann favors the professional manicure, mostly for the pampering that goes along with it. "Manicures and pedicures are a mini-getaway, a feel-good type of service," she says. "I love how many nail salons have menus now. You can get anything from a polish change to a total spa manicure, where they do your nails and your skin."

If you decide to go to a salon, assess whether the nail technician appears clean, neatly dressed, and friendly. "If you don't like what you see, walk out," Weiss-Fischmann says. "You have many other choices."

One of those, of course, is to do your nails yourself. A good manicure involves more than just slapping on a coat of paint. But with some patience and the tips in this list, you can give yourself professional looking nails.

1 BE PRUDENT WITH REMOVER
"When you take off polish, use the remover on your nail rather than all over your finger," Weiss-Fischmann says. "Because it is very drying, it can cause the skin around your nail to crack."

2 BUILD A BASE
"Always apply a base coat first," Weiss-Fischmann says. "It helps polish go on very smoothly." If your nails have ridges, use a ridge filler; if they're weak, use a nail strengthener.

3 MAKE FILING A ONE-WAY STREET

Invest in a good nail file if you don't already have one. When you use it, move the file only in one direction. That way you're less likely to break a nail, Weiss-Fischmann says.

4 HAVE FUN WITH COLOR

"With every new season and fashion trend, new nail colors are launched to complement the great looks we see on celebrities," says Jenna Hipp, the green celebrity nail stylist in Los Angeles. "For the seasons, it's fun to play with colors that mimic what's happening in nature."

Weiss-Fischmann agrees, adding that these days, anything goes in terms of color. "You go to the beach and see all of these black and blue nails," she says. "And in Fall 2009 runway shows, Chanel featured all green nails!"

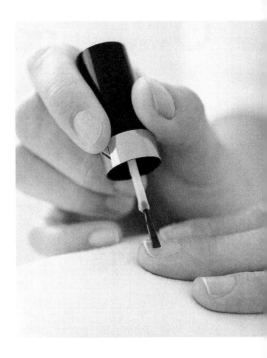

5 GO BACK FOR A TOPCOAT

"After your initial manicure, apply a topcoat of clear polish every two days," Weiss-Fischmann suggests. "It will help the polish stay on longer and restore its original luster."

6 CARE FOR YOUR CUTICLES

"Your nails look only as good as your cuticles," Hipp says. "Polish looks most professional when the cuticles are groomed and hydrated."

To keep your cuticles looking their best, apply a little cuticle softener before you get in the shower. Then as soon as you get out of the shower, push back your cuticles with your towel. Also, moisturize your cuticles twice a day with cuticle oil. If you tend to forget, Hipp suggests stashing the oil in your glove box and applying it before your morning commute and your drive home. Try Sparitual's Cuti-Cocktail or OPI's Avoplex Cuticle Oil.

7 LAY ON THE LOTION

"You don't realize how much sun your hands get, especially if you drive a lot," Weiss-Fischmann says. "There are great lotions with SPF that can help make your hands look younger." Or go a step further: Apply a hand mask to your hands and cover them with cotton gloves for a little in-home spa treatment.

your list

_____

_____

_____

_____

_____

_____

_____

6 ways to find a good day spa

mini LIST

Ask the right questions

Before you set foot in a day spa, you should ask some specific questions to make sure that it is a good fit. The following list is from James Corbett, owner of the James Corbett Studio & Spa in New York City:

- What are the theme and mission statements of the spa?

- Which product lines does the spa use? Once you know the brand names, do some research. Many establishments are offering wonderful natural and organic products in their treatments.

- What kinds of treatment packages are available? Can changes be made to standard packages to customize them?

- How many treatment rooms are available?

- What kind of education and experience do staff members have?

IN THE LAST few decades, day spas have emerged as mini-getaways for women (and some men), offering a diverse array of services from facials, manicures, and pedicures to full-body treatments. Because these facilities promote themselves as venues for complete relaxation and self-indulgence—usually at no small monetary cost—you want to find a spa where you feel comfortable and safe. Here's how.

1 DO YOUR HOMEWORK

Whether you're new to an area or just new to the world of day spas, you can start your search by asking for referrals from friends and colleagues. The Internet is another excellent resource. "Look for a spa with a website that allows you to ask questions," says hairstylist Paul Labrecque. Then you can confirm that a facility offers the service(s) you want before you even make an appointment.

2 BE WARY OF "MEDI-SPAS"

Some day spas reach outside their scope of practice, offering services that really are the domain of licensed medical professionals. "Such services—like doctor's-grade chemical peels—should be performed in a physician's office because you must be monitored afterward for swelling and other reactions," Labrecque says. "Plus, if something goes wrong, you want to make sure that someone is held accountable."

Other services to steer clear of include Botox and Restylane treatments. A good day spa will outsource these services and refer you to a reputable doctor who can administer them safely, Labrecque says.

3 SCAN FOR SPOTLESSNESS

"Personally, I would never want a facial or hair treatment done in a dirty room," Labrecque says. He suggests discreetly inspecting a facility to confirm that is clean from top to bottom, from the bathrooms and changing rooms to the brushes and bowls.

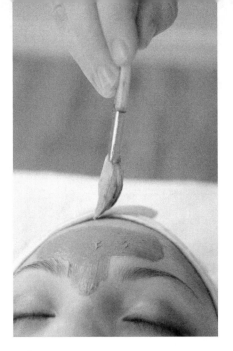

6 GIVE POINTS FOR FLEXIBILITY

When you visit a day spa, you should be the top priority. "I have never understood when a spa says 'We're all booked up,' and the place is half-empty when you go there. I hate that in restaurants, and I hate it in spas," Labrecque says. "At our spa in Manhattan, we know that things can happen to keep a client from arriving on time. If we were inflexible, we would be turning away more business than we are accepting." Look for a spa that is equally willing to accommodate a change in your schedule.

4 NOTICE HOW YOU'RE TREATED

"A day spa should engage you on every sensory level; if it doesn't, it's not worthy of the title of 'spa,'" says Shel Pink, founder of SpaRitual, a vegan body care company in Los Angeles. "Pay attention to the overall vibration and impression you get from the moment you enter a spa. If you notice an unfriendly or uninformed staff, or staff members who have an attitude or a general lack of interest in your needs, walk out."

Chances are that you're spending good money for a spa's services, so you're entitled to a good experience. "The customer is always right, and that's how you should be treated," Labrecque says.

5 SHOW LOYALTY

"Choose the spa that not only offers the kinds of products and treatments you are looking for but also has a therapist you connect with," Pink says. "When you find that person, be sure to request him or her on your next visit. Frequent appointments with the same therapist build a relationship and make him or her better able to readily address your health and wellness needs."

your list

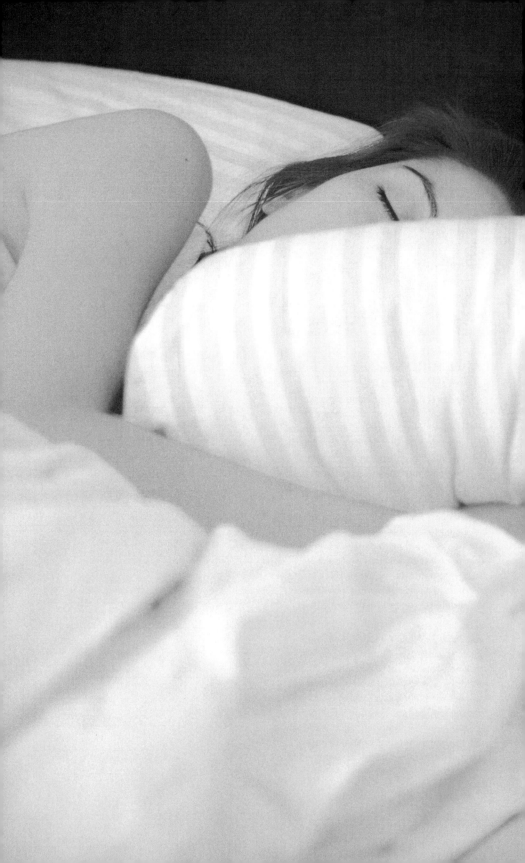

chapter 5 health

top 10 smart health moves

mini LIST

Foods to fuel a walking workout

Looking for the perfect pre- or post-walk snack? Try one of these.

1. **Coffee.** Even a small amount of caffeine (1 to 2 cups of coffee) an hour before exercising can extend your workout's duration by 50%.

2. **Granola.** Eating the whole grains generally found in granola helps to burn more fat during exercise and for 3 hours afterward, compared with eating refined grains, reports a new British study. Your granola should have no more than 7 grams of fat per serving.

3. **Chocolate milk.** Sip it after exercise. The combination of carbs and protein improves muscle recovery. Stick with low-fat or fat-free milk, and limit the chocolate syrup (2 tablespoons add 100 calories).

YOU PROBABLY WOULD agree that you have a pretty good handle on what you should be doing to stay healthy and disease-free. Still, the constant stream of new research findings can complicate your efforts to keep track of the latest dos and don'ts. With this in mind, we've asked Joyce Frye, DO, MSCE, a board-certified holistic physician and assistant professor at the Center for Integrative Medicine, University of Maryland Medical School, to assist in distilling the universe of current health information into the 10 most important self-care strategies. Be prepared for a few surprises!

1 HAVE DINNER WITH YOUR FAMILY

Conversation over the evening meal helps to maintain strong family relationships, Frye says. If you have school-age children, it's an opportunity to find out what they're up to and who they're hanging around with. And if you make dinner at home, you get to control the nutrition. As for what you eat, Frye's main advice is to minimize heavily processed foods. "Avoid anything that has ingredients with lots of syllables or that comes in a package with words you don't understand," she says.

2 PRACTICE DEEP BREATHING

Sit with your arms and legs uncrossed. Relax. Inhale deeply from your abdomen. Then exhale as much air as you can, relaxing your muscles as you do. "The exhalation phase should be longer than the inhalation phase," says Frye. "Count while you're doing your deep breathing, and whatever count you get to on the inhalation, increase that by half on the exhalation, so if your inhale is a 4 count, your exhale should be a 6 count."

3 LAUGH!

"A good, hearty laugh reduces levels of the stress hormones cortisol and epinephrine," Frye says. "Laughter also has been shown to increase the number of cells that produce antibodies and enhance the effectiveness of T-cells, an important component of the immune system." If you need something to tickle your funny bone, rent a funny movie, buy a joke book, or take in a local comedy show.

4 SAY "I LOVE YOU" TO SOMEONE

Opening up and expressing your innermost feelings is a great emotional release. "Telling someone whom you really care about how you feel about him or her pushes you to step outside of yourself and stop focusing on your own needs," Frye explains. "It helps you think about others and, ultimately, about the real purpose of life, which is to love one another and care about one another."

5 S-T-R-E-T-C-H

Stretching improves flexibility, and flexibility is analogous to homeostasis, which is the body's way of centering itself. "Flexibility in the physical sense increases flexibility in the mental sense," Frye says. She recommends stretching first thing in the morning and then throughout the day, even at work. "Everyone should stretch his or her entire body every day," she says.

6 DO THE PINCH TEST

Wondering whether you need to lose a few pounds? Try this simple test: Pinch the skin around your abdomen. If there's more than an inch of flab between your two fingers, it's too much. "Abdominal fat puts pressure on the renal arteries and raises blood pressure," Frye says. "It also increases insulin resistance and diabetes risk."

7 PARK YOUR CAR AND WALK

We could learn a lot from the Europeans, who walk everywhere. Of course, depending where you live, hoofing it to the office or supermarket may not be practical. Instead, aim for getting in a brisk walk at least three days a week. "Walking is a terrific cardio workout, and it can help you lose weight," Frye says. "Walking while listening to music will help you maintain your pace."

8 TAKE A MULTIVITAMIN

No matter how conscientious we are about our eating habits, we'll have lapses on occasion. Plus, we need to account for variations in the sources of food, the nutrients in the soil, and time for, say, our broccoli to travel from the fields to the fridge. Against all of these variables, taking a multivitamin is accessible, inexpensive insurance, Frye says. If you have trouble swallowing pills, she suggests looking for a liquid or powder multivitamin product, which you can mix into juice, oatmeal, or applesauce.

9 FLOSS YOUR TEETH

Bacteria between teeth can lead to gum disease, which in turn raises the risk of heart disease and stroke. "Studies also have shown a very clear connection between inflammation and joint disease, and periodontal disease is a major source of inflammation," Frye notes. The American Dental Association recommends flossing daily.

10 GET ENOUGH SLEEP

Adequate sleep supports immune function, sharpens your brain, slows the aging process, and lifts your spirits. So how much sleep do you need? "You know you're getting enough sleep if you can wake up spontaneously without your alarm clock," Frye says.

your list
_____
_____
_____
_____
_____
_____

6 ways to add 10 years to your life

mini LIST

Instant age erasers

Take off years in an instant with these tips.

1. Lightweight, oversize scarves can conceal your décolletage, hiding sun damage and chest wrinkles.

2. Cinching belts add shape and help carve out a waist.

3. When you're dressed in a skirt, wearing shoes that match your skin color creates the illusion of having longer legs, which slims your entire body.

4. Bangs hide trouble areas like your forehead, where fine lines will begin appearing as early as your thirties. Similarly, layered bangs (meaning they're longer on the sides) disguise eye wrinkles.

5. Lip gloss creates an illusion of fuller, plumper puckers.

WOULDN'T IT BE great if we could drive to the local drugstore and buy a bottle of Fountain of Youth? We can't, of course—at least not yet. But that doesn't mean there isn't plenty we can do to stay healthy and vital no matter how many birthdays we've celebrated. Adopt these 6 no-fail rules to give yourself the best chance of looking and feeling as young as possible for as long as possible.

1 FILL YOUR PLATE WITH COLOR

The biggest anti-aging breakthrough in recent history comes from new discoveries about the power of antioxidants. As the cells in our body metabolize oxygen, unstable molecules called free radicals form. These cause cellular damage that has been linked to heart disease and Alzheimer's. Many scientists theorize that most signs of aging are the direct result of free radicals attacking our cells. Antioxidants neutralize free radicals, preventing them from doing any damage and thereby slowing the aging process. "Antioxidants can even reverse damage to our cells," says Bonnie Taub-Dix, RD, a spokesperson for the American Dietetic Association. Research has been pointing to a strong connection between foods loaded with antioxidants and a longer, healthier life. The best food sources of these amazing nutrients easy to spot because they're bursting with color: berries, bell peppers, pomegranates, tomatoes, spinach, broccoli, and brussels sprouts.

2 RELY ON ANTIOXIDANT-RICH FOODS, NOT SUPPLEMENTS

In the massive Iowa Women's Health Survey, researchers found that of the 34,492 female participants, those who ate foods rich in the antioxidant vitamin E (such as nuts) were less likely to suffer strokes. Vitamin E in supplement form, on the other hand, provided no protection.

Natural foods—those that have been minimally processed, if at all—contain "thousands of compounds that interact in complex ways," says Frank Hu, PhD, associate professor of nutrition and epidemiology at the Harvard School of Public Health. "If you take one out, there's no predicting how it will function on its own."

3 SIP GREEN TEA

Packed with potent antioxidants called catechins, green tea may be the single most life-prolonging substance you can put in your mouth. A cup a day can reduce your chances of developing high blood pressure by 46%. Drink more, and you cut your risk by 65%.

Which green tea is best? A study in the *Journal of Food Science* found that of 77 brands tested, Stash Darjeeling organic green tea delivers the greatest number of catechins: 100 per gram.

4 BUDDY UP TO A BARBELL

Starting at about age 40, your metabolism slows by roughly 5% each decade. By age 50, you'll have lost 5 pounds of muscle and gained about 10 pounds of fat. Lifting weights counters this decline, boosting your metabolism by about 7%, which burns about 100 extra calories a day. With more muscle, you'll also have more energy to get back into the fat-burning physical activities you enjoy.

Be sure to check with your physician before beginning any exercise program. Plan for three strength-training sessions a week, with each lasting about 20 minutes. Start with 5- to 10-pound dumbbells. If you're lifting the weights easily at the end of each set, switch to heavier weights. Work your way to three sets of 10 reps. For barbell workouts and videos, visit prevention.com/health/fitness/strength-training.

5 INCORPORATE CARDIO

To fight middle-age spread, engage in heart-pumping, calorie-burning cardiovascular activity six days a week. If you belong to the gym, try the step machine or elliptical trainer. Depending on the activity, you'll burn about 450 calories in 25 to 50 minutes. As your fitness level increases, you can challenge yourself by making at least two of your weekly cardio

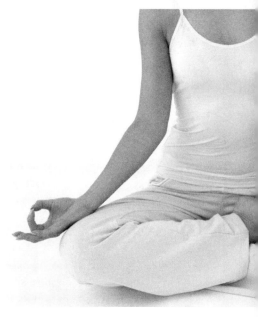

workouts an interval routine, alternating bursts of intensity and recovery.

6 STRIKE A (YOGA) POSE

Stress is among the biggest contributors to the aging process, robbing you of precious sleep, increasing harmful inflammation, even damaging your DNA. Recent research has shown that yoga reduces markers of oxidative stress, a condition that can accelerate the cellular damage linked to aging. Daily yoga practice carries a greater benefit than a weekly class because you're fighting stress a little at a time, says Carol Krucoff, a yoga therapist for Duke Integrative Medicine at Duke University and creator of the CD *Healing Moves Yoga*.

your list

_____

_____

_____

_____

_____

_____

7 ways to shorten your lifespan

my favorite...
Stress-Busting Technique

Cynthia Paige, MD, assistant professor at New Jersey Medical School

"My favorite stress-busting technique is to take a daily vacation," Paige says. "I carve out a few minutes each day to get very calm and relaxed. If it's a sunny day, I notice the blue sky. If it's raining, I step outside and smell the fresh air that you can only experience after a rain. I think about the bountiful blessings in my life. After just a few minutes of this reframing, I feel centered again."

IN AN EPISODE of *Laverne & Shirley*, health-conscious Shirley announces to Laverne, "I treat my body like a temple. You treat *yours* like an amusement park!" Life is all about choices. You can choose to hold on to your youth, but it takes strategy and commitment to a healthy lifestyle. And if any of the following are part of your current repertoire, you may need to rethink your aging ways.

1 SMOKING
Smoking is a major factor in the three leading causes of death in the United States: cardiovascular disease, cancer, and stroke. It also contributes to disease in just about every organ system of the human body. "For every death from smoking, there are about 20 causes of non-fatal disease that are associated with smoking," says Cynthia Paige, MD, assistant professor in the Department of Family Medicine, University of Medicine & Dentistry of New Jersey, New Jersey Medical School.

2 OBESITY
Studies have shown that obesity can take about 13 years off of a person's life. Every organ system is impacted by diseases that accompany obesity, such as diabetes, hypertension, and high cholesterol. To slim down, Paige suggests limiting processed and fast foods, which are calorie-rich and nutrient-poor.

3 A LOW-FIBER DIET
"Fiber helps to lower cholesterol and improve digestion by increasing transit time," Paige says. "Increased transit time through the intestines has been associated with a lower risk of colon cancer." Another benefit of foods high in fiber is that they tend to not be high in fat, salt, or sugar. Good sources of fiber include vegetables, fruits, nuts, and grains.

4 SOCIAL ISOLATION

A 10-year study of older populations in South Australia, recently published in the *Journal of Epidemiology and Community Health*, concluded that people with friends and confidants have longer life expectancies.

Friends can be positive influences, helping us to stop smoking and encouraging us to exercise. They also keep us from becoming isolated as we get older, the study authors wrote. "We know that isolation increases the risk of depression, which can result in a decreased life span," Paige notes. So make time for your friends by scheduling lunches, phone calls, or evenings out—whatever keeps you in touch with your social circle.

5 PESSIMISM

Several studies that have tracked octogenarians determined that optimism and a positive outlook are life-preserving, Paige says. A negative attitude, on the other hand, often goes hand-in-hand with depression—and depression can shorten life expectancy. According to recent research conducted at McGill University and the University of Toronto, stroke patients who were most apathetic had the lowest rates of recovery.

A great way to cultivate your inner optimist is to spend time involved in activities that encourage positivity, such as volunteering. For more tips, see page 82.

6 STRESS

"We know that being under stress, and not recognizing and doing anything to reduce that stress, increases the risk of cardiovascular disease and death," Paige says. "Research also shows that stress inhibits the immune system, which leaves us more vulnerable to cancer and infection, among other diseases."

7 ANGER

In studies that tracked people who'd suffered heart attacks, those who remained angry fared worse and did not live as long as those who were more forgiving. "That high-stress type A personality contributes to high rates of heart disease and high blood pressure," Paige says. "It also raises blood sugar and interferes with a person's ability to heal from disease."

your list

5 facts to flu-proof your body

mini LIST

Hand-washing essentials

Keeping your hands clean is one of the most important steps you can take to avoid getting sick and spreading germs to other people. Here's how to do it right.

1. Wet your hands with clean running water—warm, if possible. Apply soap.

2. Rub your hands together to make a lather. Scrub all surfaces and under your fingernails.

3. Continue rubbing your hands for 20 seconds. To keep track of the time, imagine singing, "Happy Birthday" twice through.

4. Rinse your hands thoroughly under running water.

5. Dry your hands using a paper towel—yes, even at home. If you prefer to use hand towels from your bath, be sure to launder them regularly.

YOU CAN TELL when flu season rolls around. One minute you're having a delightful lunch with friends. But as soon as one of them coughs, you begin to eye them with an air of suspicion—and wonder how long you have before you're coughing, too.

Although the flu is quite common, it isn't to be taken lightly. The Centers for Disease Control and Prevention report that more than 200,000 people are hospitalized with flu complications each year, and about 36,000 die from it. "Flu comes on suddenly, and the symptoms are much worse than a cold," notes Christopher Czaja, MD, infection control officer for the National Jewish Health Hospital in Denver. Typical symptoms—which last about 5 days—include fever, chills, muscle aches, runny nose, cough, headache, fatigue, and sore throat.

To limit your chances of infection with the influenza virus, heed this advice.

1 GET THE VACCINE

Although no vaccine is 100% effective in preventing disease, vaccination is the primary method of flu prevention. "Children under age 5, those with chronic medical conditions, and the elderly are at higher risk than the general population for serious complications from the flu," Czaja notes. "Vaccinating these groups is critical." Autumn is the best time to get vaccinated, although winter isn't too late, as flu outbreaks sometimes continue into early spring.

The vaccine can be administered via injection or as a nasal spray. Despite conventional wisdom, you can't get flu from the vaccine. However, the vaccine does contain small amounts of the weakened influenza virus and some people experience mild fever, body aches, and fatigue for a few days after receiving the injection, along with soreness at the injection site. For the nasal vaccine, the most common side effect is runny nose and/or congestion.

2 SCRUB UP

"Wash your hands often to avoid getting sick," Czaja says. "And urge everyone who lives and works with you to wash their hands, too, to stop the spread of

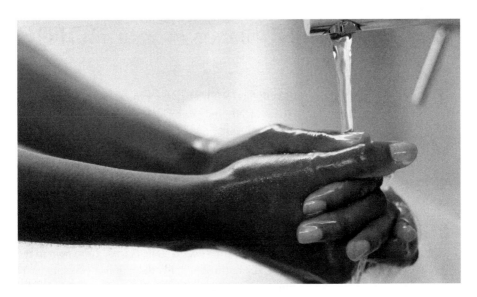

infection." Keep a bottle of alcohol-based hand sanitizer in your car or purse, so you can clean your hands after shopping, eating, or running errands. If you are concerned about killing the healthy bacteria on your hands, stick to plain old soap and water—and keep a good moisturizer around to prevent your skin from chapping.

3 SNUFF THE BUTTS

If you smoke, quit. If you don't, avoid establishments that permit smoking and people who smoke. All that smoke can aggravate respiratory symptoms, increasing your risk of flu infection, Czaja says.

4 BE CAREFUL OF THE COMPANY YOU KEEP

Always avoid situations in which you'd be in close contact with someone who has the flu, a cold, or bronchitis, Czaja advises. "If someone is showing symptoms, now is not the best time to visit," he says.

5 DRINK BLACK TEA

Drinking 5 cups a day for 2 weeks can turn your immune system's T cells into "Hulk cells" that produce 10 times more interferon, a protein that battles cold and flu infections, according to a Harvard study. Don't like black tea? The green variety will also do the trick. If you can't stomach drinking that much, you can still get added protection with fewer cups.

your list

7 germiest places in your home

facts & figures

50
thousand

Number of bacteria on the average kitchen sink. That's about 1,000 times the number on the average toilet.

IF YOU THINK it's healthier to eat your meals in your kitchen than your *bathroom*, we have news for you. When microbiologists at the University of Arizona ranked household areas by their germ load, the kitchen took dubious top honors. "In most homes, you're better off eating off the toilet than the kitchen counter," says Charles P. Gerba, PhD, one of the microbiologists and a leading hygiene researcher. "People tend to use antibacterial products in the bathroom but not in the kitchen."

Although the kitchen is the biggest germ pool in the house, the bathroom holds the number-two spot (pardon the pun). According to Gerba's research, the sink, faucet, and shower drain can harbor bacteria that cause diarrhea and infection.

Before you invest in a hazmat suit, there are many simpler things that you can do to clean up the germiest places in your home.

1 ZAP THE KITCHEN SPONGE

Those tiny crevices trap bacteria, so when you wipe up with a sponge, you're actually spreading germs all over the place. You can kill those microbes by microwaving your wet sponge or running it through the dishwasher daily.

Even better: Instead of sponging surfaces, spritz the sink, countertops, and cutting boards with an antimicrobial spray after each meal. Let it set (the product label should say for how long) before wiping it up with a damp paper towel. These sprays are often multi-purpose, so look on the label to make sure it specifies use in the kitchen and on countertops.

If you're concerned about the environment, use paper towels made from 100% recycled paper (minimum 80% post-consumer) or used, clean rags. Keep on hand a stack of terrycloth rags ripped from worn bath towels (about 10 inches square). When done with a task, wash them with hot water and line dry (sunshine also kills germs and helps fade stains).

2 SANITIZE DISH TOWELS

In a recent study involving hundreds of homes across the United States, about 7% of kitchen towels were contaminated with MRSA (methicillin-resistant *Staphylococcus aureus*), the difficult-to-treat staph bacteria that can cause life-threatening skin infections. Dish towels also rated tops for dangerous strains of *Escherichia coli* and other bacteria. Save the dish rag to dry just-washed pots and plates. Change towels or launder at least twice a week in hot water and bleach.

3 DISINFECT THE DISPOSAL

That raw chicken or spinach that you're rinsing off in the kitchen sink could be loaded with harmful bacteria. Although the metal part of a garbage disposal produces ions that can help kill the germs, they still love to grow on the crevices in and around the slimy rubber stopper. That means your disposal can become party central for bacteria, contaminating whatever touches it—dishes, utensils, even your hands. At least once a week, clean the disposal's rubber stopper with a diluted bleach solution (follow the directions on the bleach label); soap and water aren't enough.

4 CLEAN THE FAUCET SCREEN

It may surprise you to learn that the metal aeration screen at the tip of the kitchen faucet is a total germ magnet. Running water keeps the screen moist, creating an ideal environment for bacterial growth. If you accidentally touch the screen with dirty fingers or food, the bacteria can take up residence inside the faucet, explains Kelly Reynolds, PhD, a microbiologist and associate professor of community environment and policy at the University of Arizona College of Public Health. Over time, the bacteria build up and form a wall of pathogens called a biofilm that sticks to the screen. "Eventually, that biofilm may become big enough to break off and get onto your food or dishes," Reynolds notes.

An easy fix: Once a week, remove the screen and soak it in a diluted bleach solution (follow the directions on the bleach label). Replace the screen, and let the water run a few minutes before using.

5 DE-BUG BATHROOM FIXTURES

In the bathroom, wipe down the sink, faucet, shower drain, and toilet seat with an antimicrobial cleaner once a week. This is especially important if someone in your home has a cold, the flu, or an intestinal illness. It's fine to use disposable tow-elettes, such as Clorox Disinfecting Wipes, if a quick cleanup is needed.

6 SQUIRT THE SHOWER

Use an after-shower disinfecting spray regularly to prevent buildup of mold, mildew, and grime. After each shower or bath, lightly mist the entire area, including the inside of the curtain or shower door. No need to rinse or wipe off.

7 DON'T IGNORE THE BATHROOM FLOOR

Be sure to mop the floor—including behind the commode—every two weeks. An extendable cleaning tool (like a Swiffer) makes it easier to get into any tight spots.

your list

7 germiest public places

mini LIST

Doctor's office savvy

A doctor's office is not the place to be if you're trying to avoid germs. These tips can help limit your exposure.

1. Take your own books and magazines (and kid's toys, if you have your children or grandchildren with you).

2. Also pack your own tissues and hand sanitizers, which should be at least 60% alcohol content.

3. In the waiting room, leave at least two chairs between you and the other patients to reduce your chances of picking up their bugs. Germ droplets from coughing and sneezing can travel about 3 feet before falling to the floor.

AN AVERAGE ADULT can touch as many as 30 objects within a minute, including germ-harboring, high-traffic surfaces such as light switches, doorknobs, phone receivers, and remote controls. At home, you do all that you can to keep the germs at bay. But what happens when you step out the door to go to dinner, do some grocery shopping, or visit the doctor's office? Know where germs are most likely to lurk, as you'll find out here.

1 RESTAURANT MENUS

Have you ever seen anyone wash off a menu? Probably not. A recent study in the *Journal of Medical Virology* reported that cold and flu viruses can survive for 18 hours on hard surfaces. If it's a popular restaurant, hundreds of people could be handling the menus—and passing their germs on to you. Never let a menu touch your plate or silverware, and wash your hands after you place your order.

2 LEMON WEDGES

According to a 2007 study in the *Journal of Environmental Health*, nearly 70% of the lemon wedges perched on the rims of restaurant glasses contain disease-causing microbes. When the researchers ordered drinks at 21 different restaurants, they found 25 different microorganisms lingering on the 76 lemons that they secured, including *E. coli* and other fecal bacteria. Tell your server that you'd prefer your beverage sans fruit. Why risk it?

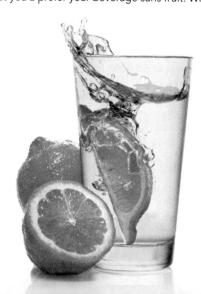

3 CONDIMENT DISPENSERS

It's the rare eatery that regularly bleaches its condiment containers. And the reality is that many people don't wash their hands before eating, says Kelly Reynolds, PhD. So while you may be diligent, the guy who poured the ketchup before you may not have been, which means his germs are now on your fries. Squirt hand sanitizer on the outside of the condiment bottle or use a disinfectant wipe before you grab it. Holding the bottle with a napkin won't help; napkins are porous, so microorganisms can pass right through, Reynolds says.

4 RESTROOM DOOR HANDLES

Don't think you can escape the restroom without touching the door handle? Palm a spare paper towel after you wash up and use it to grasp the handle. Yes, other patrons may think you're a germ-phobe—but you'll never see them again, and you're the one who won't get sick.

5 SOAP DISPENSERS

About 25% of public restroom dispensers are contaminated with fecal bacteria. Soap that harbors bacteria may seem ironic, but that's exactly what a recent study found. "Most of these containers are never cleaned, so bacteria grow as the soap scum builds up," says Charles Gerba, PhD. "And the bottoms are touched by dirty hands, so there's a continuous culture feeding millions of bacteria." Be sure to scrub hands thoroughly with plenty of hot water for 15 to 20 seconds—and if you happen to have an alcohol-based hand sanitizer, use that, too.

6 GROCERY CARTS

The handles of almost two-thirds of the shopping carts tested in a 2007 study at the University of Arizona were contaminated with fecal bacteria. In fact, the bacterial counts of the carts exceeded those of the average public restroom. Swab the handle with a disinfectant wipe before grabbing hold (stores are starting to provide them, so look around for a dispenser). And while you're wheeling around the supermarket, skip the free food samples, which are nothing more than communal hand-to-germ-to-mouth zones.

7 AIRPLANE BATHROOMS

When Gerba tested for microbes in the bathrooms of commercial jets, he found surfaces from faucets to doorknobs to be contaminated with *E. coli*. It's not surprising, then, that you're 100 times more likely to catch a cold when you're airborne, according to a recent study in the *Journal of Environmental Health Research*. To protect yourself, try taking green tea supplements. In a 2007 study from the University of Florida, people who took a 450-milligram green tea supplement twice a day for 3 months had one-third fewer days of cold symptoms. The supplement brand used in the study was Immune Guard ($30 for 60 pills; immune-guard.us).

your list

5 tips to protect your heart

30 percent

How much you can cut your cardiovascular disease risk if you become physically active, according to the American Heart Association.

THE CURRENT STATISTICS on heart disease are as sobering as ever. Consider:

- Heart disease ranks as the number one cause of death in the US.
- Almost one-third of women have some form of heart disease, and most don't realize it.
- Half of the men who die suddenly from heart disease had no prior symptoms.

But there is good news. According to the latest research, you can lower your heart disease risk just by making some simple lifestyle changes. But you need to start now. "It's important to take care of your heart before you have any symptoms," says Arthur Agatston, MD, a Miami cardiologist and author of *The South Beach Diet Heart Program*. Here's what to do.

1 TALK TO YOUR MOM

According to a 2006 Swedish study, your heart disease risk spikes by 43% if your mother is affected. This may be more environmental than genetic, since children typically spend more time with their mothers and tend to learn lifestyle habits from them. But even if you exercise and don't smoke, your risk could be as much as 82% higher if both of your parents have heart disease.

Depending on your family history, Agatston recommends several in-depth tests that go beyond the normal blood workup every few years, starting in your mid-forties. Talk to your doctor about the following: a 64-slice computed tomography (CT) scan of the heart; a standard lipid profile; a C-reactive Protein (CRP) test; a homocysteine blood test; an exercise stress test; a thallium stress test, and an angiogram.

2 DON'T FEAR MEDICATION

If a blood test shows that your cholesterol is high, lifestyle changes—in the form of diet and exercise—might help. But by themselves, they may not be enough. In that case, your doctor may prescribe a cholesterol-reducing medication known as a statin, which keeps the liver from

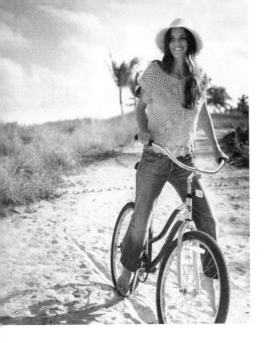

fatty fish such as wild (not farmed) salmon, tuna, and sardines.

The American Heart Association (AHA) recommends that no more than 7% of your daily calories come from saturated fats such as red meat, butter, and full-fat dairy products like whole milk and cheese. Further, only 1% of your daily calories should be in the form of trans fats, found mostly in processed foods like cookies, crackers, and potato chips.

5 MOVE YOUR BODY
According to a 2010 AHA survey, although 58% of American adults resolved to make improvements in their health, more than half also said that they often find reasons not to exercise, ranging from too much stress at work to having nothing to wear to simple procrastination. But here's why you should exercise: Once you become physically active, you can cut your heart disease risk by 30%. The AHA recommends engaging 150 minutes of moderate-intensity physical activity, such as brisk walking, each week. Other beneficial activities include aerobic dance, bicycling, jogging, swimming, and skiing.

producing too much cholesterol. "Statins are incredible tools in lowering cholesterol and can keep many people from suffering heart attacks," Agatston says. "But there's no question: They're meant to work together with proper diet and exercise."

3 BANISH BELLY FAT
Recent studies indicate that abdominal fat is metabolically different from other body fat. As you gain padding around your middle, the individual fat cells swell. Their size is linked to higher triglyceride levels and lower levels of HDL, the "good" cholesterol. New research from Wake Forest University Baptist Medical Center shows that the combination of diet and exercise can reduce the size of abdominal fat cells. That doesn't happen if you lose weight through diet alone.

4 INCREASE YOUR FISH CONSUMPTION
Nieca Goldberg, MD, a New York City cardiologist and author of *The Women's Healthy Heart Program*, touts the benefits of foods rich in omega-3 fatty acids. These beneficial fats may help lower blood pressure and the risk of abnormal heart rhythms. The best sources of omega-3s are

your list

8 ways to lower your cancer risk

mini LIST

Cancer-fighting foods

Be sure to stock up on these nutrients to pack a powerful anti-cancer punch:

1. **Selenium:** 55 micrograms a day. *Food sources:* Brazil nuts, snapper, and shrimp.

2. **Carotenoids:** 2,310 IU a day. *Food sources:* carrots and butternut squash.

3. **Vitamin E:** 55 micrograms a day. *Food sources:* sunflower seeds, hazlenuts, and peanut butter.

4. **Isothiocyanates:** No recommended daily intake. *Food sources:* broccoli, brussels sprouts, and cauliflower.

5. **Calcium:** 1,200 milligrams a day. *Food sources:* milk, yogurt, Swiss cheese, kale, broccoli, bok choy, collard greens, and spinach.

AN ANCIENT CHINESE proverb cautions, "Fortune and disaster do not come through gates, but man himself invites their arrival." Science bears out the disaster part: One-third of all cancer deaths are related to lifestyle, according to the American Cancer Society (ACS). Here's how to reduce your risk.

1 LOWER YOUR BMI

A recent study found that women who gained 60 pounds after age 18 were up to three times more likely to be diagnosed with breast cancer. Being overweight or obese is a risk factor for several other cancers, including those of the colon, endometrium, esophagus, and kidney. As the ACS explains, excess weight causes the body to produce and circulate more of the hormones estrogen and insulin, which can stimulate cancer growth. To reduce your cancer risk, aim for a BMI below 25.

2 ENGAGE IN EXERCISE

Increasing the amount of physical activity that you do not only helps melt away extra pounds, it also boosts your immune function and lowers estrogen levels—both of which have protective effects. It's best to get 45 to 60 minutes of heart-pumping activity most days of the week, but even a moderate level of exercise (30 minutes a day, 5 days a week) can make a difference.

3 TAKE VITAMIN D

It's a triple threat: Vitamin D encourages the death of abnormal cells, improves immunity, and stops the growth of blood vessels that nourish tumors, says researcher William Grant, PhD. One study found that those who got at least 600 IU of vitamin D every day were 41% less likely to develop pancreatic cancer than those who got less than 150 IU.

Your body can make all of the vitamin D that it needs with help from the sun's rays. Though excessive sun exposure can increase skin cancer risk, a growing number of experts believe that a modest amount of sun time—about 10 minutes a day—outweighs the risk by replenishing vitamin D stores. Food sources of vitamin D include fortified milk and orange juice, yogurt, cereals, egg yolks, and fish such as salmon and tuna.

4 EAT A RAINBOW OF FOODS

Get at least 5 servings of fruits and vegetables each day, especially those with the most vibrant colors—an indicator of high antioxidant content. Antioxidant nutrients work together to protect against many types of cancer, including lung, mouth, esophagus, stomach, and colon cancers.

5 SHRINK THAT STEAK

When researchers examined dietary data collected from nearly 280,000 men and 190,000 women, they found a link between the consumption of red meat and an increased risk of lung cancer in both men (22%) and women (13%). Limit the red meat in your diet, and keep the portion to no more than 3 ounces (about the size of a deck of cards.)

6 SCHEDULE A MAMMOGRAM

Aside from non-melanoma skin cancer, breast cancer is the most commonly diagnosed cancer among women. The ACS recommends yearly mammograms starting at age 40. If you're in your forties, ask for a digital mammogram, which does a better job for younger women with dense breasts. In a large, multicenter study, digital scans found 15% more cancers than standard mammograms in women under age 50. Women at high risk for breast cancer should have annual mammograms, along with MRIs, starting either at age 30 or at an age determined by a physician.

7 ASK ABOUT PREVENTIVES

If you are in your sixties or you have a family history of breast cancer, talk to your doctor about tamoxifen, raloxifene, and similar preventive medications. Tamoxifen has been shown to slash breast cancer by 50% in women at high risk for the disease, according to the National Women's Health Resource Center.

8 REDUCE "ELECTROSMOG"

Recent research has identified a link between electromagnetic fields (EMFs) and increased cancer risk. Sources of EMFs include cell phones, cordless phones, cell phone towers, and electrical power lines. To minimize your exposure, use landline phones whenever possible, keep your laptop off your lap, and unplug any electronic gadgets that you aren't using.

Also, avoid using Bluetooth headsets. Contrary to popular belief, when combined with a cell phone, even these headsets can exceed current safety limits.

your list

5 ways to lower your diabetes risk

mini LIST

Eat to beat diabetes

To help balance your blood sugar—and shed pounds, too—add the following foods to your shopping list:

1. **Goji berries.** Scientists have discovered that the sugars responsible for the sweetness of goji berries also reduce insulin resistance in laboratory rats. Look for juice blends featuring goji berries in your local grocery store.

2. **Fat-free yogurt.** According to a landmark Tufts–New England Medical Center study, calcium-rich foods may enhance cellular insulin response, meaning that cells use insulin more efficiently.

3. **Salmon.** This heart-healthy fish is a good source of calcium, vitamin D, and omega-3 fatty acids—all of which can help lower diabetes risk.

DID YOU KNOW that every 20 seconds, someone is diagnosed with diabetes? More than 24 million Americans already have some form of the disease, while another 57 million have prediabetes. But not all the statistics are scary; in fact, some are motivational. For example, eating just two extra servings of whole grains every day could reduce your risk by 21%. Here are more ways to keep diabetes at bay.

1 NUDGE THE SCALE

If you weigh more than you should, losing those extra pounds is one of the best things that you can do to improve your blood sugar and lower your chances of developing diabetes. And you needn't lose much to make a difference. In one study, people who were extremely overweight were 70% less likely to develop diabetes after dropping just 5% of their weight—even if they didn't exercise.

2 BYPASS THE DRIVE-THROUGH

An occasional fast-food splurge might be ok, but become a regular "fast-feeder," and your diabetes risk skyrockets. That's what University of Minnesota researchers found when they tracked 3,000 people, ages 18 to 30, for 15 years. At the start of the study, everyone was of normal weight. But those who ate fast food more than twice a week gained 10 more pounds and showed twice the rate of insulin resistance—the two major risk factors for type 2 diabetes—compared to those who indulged less than once a week.

To help take the edge off hunger when you're running errands or chauffeuring the kids, keep a bag of low-calorie trail mix in your purse or car. It will tide you over until you get home—and as a bonus, nuts can help lower blood sugar.

3 HIT THE SLEEP SWEET SPOT

A Yale University study involving 1,709 men found that those who regularly got less than 6 hours of shut-eye doubled their diabetes risk, while those who slept more than 8 hours tripled their odds. Previous research involving women has produced similar findings. "When you sleep too little or too long, because of sleep apnea, your nervous system stays on alert," explains lead researcher Klar Yaggi, MD. This interferes with hormones that regulate blood sugar. For a good night's rest, avoid caffeine (including chocolate) after noon, leave work at the office, and skip late-night TV. Oversleeping may be a sign of depression or a treatable sleep disorder, so talk with your doctor.

4 SPICE UP YOUR LIFE

German researchers enlisted 65 adults with type 2 diabetes, who took a capsule containing the equivalent of 1 gram of cinnamon powder or a placebo three times a day for 4 months. By the end of the study, those in the cinnamon group had lowered their blood sugar by about 10%, compared to 4% among the placebo users. Certain compounds in cinnamon may activate enzymes that stimulate insulin receptors. The sweet spice also has been shown to help lower cholesterol and triglycerides, blood fats that may contribute to blood sugar trouble.

5 UNWIND EVERY DAY

When you're stressed, your body is primed to take action. Your heart beats faster, your breath quickens—and your blood sugar levels skyrocket. "Under stress, your body goes into fight-or-flight mode, raising blood sugar levels in preparation to take action," explains Richard Surwit, PhD, author of *The Mind-Body Diabetes Revolution*. If your cells are insulin-resistant, the sugar builds up in your blood with nowhere to go, leading to chronically high levels.

Simple relaxation techniques can help you regain control of your stress response—and your blood sugar.

- Start your day with yoga, meditation, or a walk.
- Take three slow, deep breaths before answering the phone, when waiting in line at the bank, or while doing any potentially stress-inducing activity.
- Reclaim your Sundays as rest or fun time with family and friends, rather than using them to do housework or run errands.

(For more de-stressing strategies, see page 70).

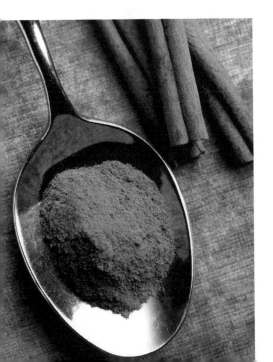

your list

7 pains you shouldn't ignore

mini LIST

Know the symptoms of a stroke

Stroke is the third leading cause of death in the United States and a leading cause of serious disability, according to the American Heart Association. If you or someone close to you is experiencing any of these symptoms, immediately call 9-1-1.

- Sudden numbness or weakness of the face, arm or leg, especially on one side of the body
- Sudden confusion, trouble speaking or understanding
- Sudden trouble seeing in one or both eyes
- Sudden trouble walking, dizziness, loss of balance or coordination
- Sudden, severe headache with no known cause

USUALLY A HEADACHE is just a headache, and heartburn is nothing more than a sign that you rang the Taco Bell once too often. Except when they're not.

Pain is your body's way of telling you that something isn't quite right. More often than not, you have some idea of what's behind it. But when it comes on suddenly, lingers longer than usual, or just seems different, it calls for medical attention—and the sooner, the better. According to our experts, all of the following pain conditions should be considered red flags

1 CHEST PAIN

"If patients were to become well versed in what I think of as the subtle language of the heart, many could avoid needless worry and expense," notes Arthur Agatston, MD, a preventive cardiologist. "Studies have found that women experience a wider range of heart attack symptoms than men do." In Agatston's experience, there are three good indicators that something isn't right, and they can occur in either gender. They are chest pain that doesn't go away, varied shortness of breath, and any upper body pain that hasn't occurred before. If you experience any of these symptoms, he says, you should call your doctor or 911 immediately.

2 SEVERE HEAD PAIN

Chances are, it's a migraine. But if it isn't accompanied by other migraine symptoms (such as a visual aura), sudden, severe head pain can signal a brain aneurysm. "A burst aneurysm can cause brain damage within minutes, so you need to call 911 immediately," advises Elsa-Grace Giardina, MD, a cardiologist and director of the Center for Women's Health at New York–Presbyterian Hospital/Columbia University Medical Center.

3 A THROBBING TOOTH

It's likely that the tooth's nerve has become damaged, probably because the surrounding pearly white enamel is cracked or rotting away. Unless you get it patched up quickly, bacteria in your mouth can invade the nerve. And you definitely don't want that breeding colony to spread throughout your body, says Kimberly Harms, DDS, a dentist outside St. Paul, Minnesota. If your tooth is already infected, you'll require a root canal, in which the tooth's bacteria-laden pulp is removed and replaced with plastic caulking material.

4 SHARP PAIN IN YOUR SIDE

You may just need some Beano. But if you feel as if you're being skewered in your right side, and you're also nauseated and running a fever, you could have appendicitis. For women, another possibility is an ovarian cyst. Typically these fluid-filled sacs are harmless and disappear on their own. But if one twists or ruptures, it can cause terrible pain.

In both cases, you're looking at emergency surgery. "If you don't remove an inflamed appendix, it can burst," says Lin Chang, MD, a gastroenterologist and co-director of the Center for Neurovisceral Sciences and Women's Health at UCLA. A twisted cyst also needs to be removed right away, as it can block blood flow to the ovary within hours.

5 ABDOMINAL DISCOMFORT WITH GAS OR BLOATING

For the past month, you've felt gassy and bloated more days than not, and it takes fewer slices of pizza to fill you up than it once did. If the symptoms are new, the worst-case scenario is ovarian cancer. In 2007, the Gynecologic Cancer Foundation released the first national consensus on early symptoms of this form of cancer: bloating, pelvic or abdominal pain, and difficulty eating. If you start experiencing them almost daily for more than two or three weeks, consider it a red flag. Schedule an appointment with your ob-gyn to discuss your symptoms.

6 BACK PAIN WITH TINGLING TOES

If you've just helped your cousin move into her new fourth-floor apartment, anti-inflammatories should banish the pain. But if they don't work, hobble to an orthopedist. "One of your discs (the spongy rings that cushion the bones in your spine) could be pressing on the spinal nerve," says Letha Griffin, MD, an orthopedist and sports medicine specialist in Atlanta. Without proper attention, you risk permanent nerve damage.

7 LEG PAIN WITH SWELLING

Your calf is extremely tender in one location, noticeably swollen, and red or warm to the touch. You might have deep-vein thrombosis (DVT), commonly known as a blood clot. Resist the urge to massage the area or to try walking off the pain. If the clot breaks free, it can travel through your veins up to your lungs and cut off your oxygen supply. Instead, see your doctor right away. He or she will do a CT scan or ultrasound to check for a DVT. If that's what you have, you'll need to take blood thinners—sometimes for up to a year—to dissolve it, says Suzanne Steinbaum, MD, director of women and heart disease for the Heart and Vascular Institute at Lenox Hill Hospital in New York City.

your list

7 must-haves for your medicine chest

mini LIST

Nature's medicine chest

Gayle Eversole, PhD, ND, recommends these natural remedies in a pinch:

1. **Cayenne powder.** Just a little cayenne powder mixed with hot water can help clear chest congestion and relieve cold and flu symptoms.

2. **Lavender or tea tree oil.** Both of these oils have antiviral, antibacterial, and antifungal properties. Use either one to soothe scrapes and burns, as well as to reduce the stinging and swelling of bug bites. Apply the undiluted oil directly to the skin.

3. **Ginger.** Ginger is great for just about any gastrointestinal symptoms. Make a tea by steeping a tablespoon of ground fresh ginger in hot water for 10 minutes, then straining and allowing to cool before drinking.

MOST OF US stock our medicine chests on an as-needed basis. But for life's minor maladies and mishaps, it's a good idea to have at least a few essentials on hand. We asked Heather Free, PharmD, spokesperson for the American Pharmacists Association, what she would recommend keeping on hand. Here's her list of must-haves.

1 FIRST AID KIT

Your kit should include alcohol swabs, burn cream, antibiotic ointment, gloves, gauze pads, tweezers, and adhesive bandages in several sizes. Free recommends checking your kit regularly to make sure that the items with expiration dates are still good. "I check mine twice each year, once in the fall and once during spring cleaning," she says.

2 THERMOMETER

Most thermometers available today are digital and run on batteries. So as with your first-aid kit, you'll need to check your thermometer periodically to make sure that it's still working. "I write the date that I put in the battery right on the battery itself, with a felt-tip pen," Free says. "I also buy spare thermometer batteries and store them all in the same spot."

To get the most accurate reading, place the thermometer under the tongue to the side of your mouth, rather than at the front. "The pockets on the side are closer to blood vessels that more accurately reflect the body's core temperature," Free explains.

Note that a temperature higher than 101°F that lasts for more than 3 days or fails to respond to treatment requires prompt medical attention.

3 ANTIHISTAMINE

Perhaps the best known of the antihistamines is Benadryl, although other brands are available. Choose one that has diphenhydramine as its active ingredient. "These products alleviate allergic symptoms such as sneezing, runny nose, and itchy or watery eyes," Free says. "They're also great for rashes and mosquito bites."

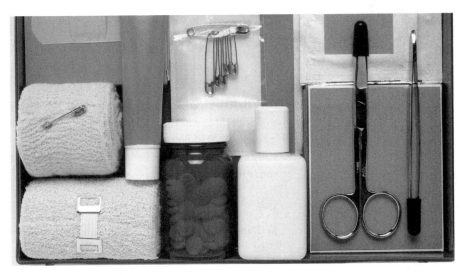

4 PEPTO-BISMOL AND GAS-X

Both of these products target gastrointestinal discomfort, Free says. Pepto-Bismol treats indigestion, upset stomach, and diarrhea, although it isn't appropriate for children under age 12. Gas-X helps to relieve the gas and pressure that may occur after a meal or with gastrointestinal illness.

5 PAIN RELIEVERS

Acetaminophen relieves mild pain and also helps to lower fever. What it can't do is reduce inflammation, as aspirin and NSAIDs such as ibuprofen and naproxen can. Free cautions that aspirin should not be given to children under age 12 because of the risk of Reye syndrome.

6 HYDROCORTISONE CREAM

"This steroid cream can be applied to minor rashes caused by poisonous plants such as poison ivy and poison oak," Free says. "It reduces pain, redness, and swelling. It's also great for soothing sunburn and razor bumps."

7 ANTIFUNGAL CREAM OR GEL

Fungal infections live on the skin and breed best in warm, moist conditions such as locker rooms, pools, and bathrooms. Look for a product containing miconazole, tolnaftate, or clotrimazole. "These products treat athlete's foot and nail fungus," Free notes.

your list

10 natural remedies that work

mini **LIST**

7 super spices

New research from the University of Georgia reveals that antioxidant-rich herbs and spices can block the formation of harmful compounds associated with aging. Here are the top seven spices from the study.

1. **Ground cloves.** Mix into cake dough for spicy sweetness.

2. **Ground Jamaican allspice.** Add to lean ground beef when making hamburgers.

3. **Sage.** Try it in your favorite tomato sauce.

4. **Marjoram.** Steep in hot water to make an herbal tea.

5. **Ground cinnamon.** Sprinkle on whole wheat toast drizzled with honey.

6. **Ground oregano.** Use to top homemade garlic bread or pizza.

7. **Thyme.** Stir into scrambled eggs for a fragrant flavor boost.

YOUR BODY CAN throw you a curve at any time. Depending on the nature of the problem, you may be able to self-treat at home, using remedies that you may already have on hand—not in your medicine chest, but in your kitchen. Try one of these in a pinch.

1 GINGER

Ginger is the go-to remedy for nausea; it's especially effective for morning sickness. Make a batch of frozen ginger chips so that they're ready when you need them. Here's how: Infuse fresh ginger in hot water. Strain, then freeze the tea in ice cube trays. Crush the cubes and suck the icy chips throughout the day for gentle relief.

2 SUGAR

To stifle hiccups, swallow 1 to 2 teaspoons of sugar. The dry granules stimulate and reset the irritated nerve that is causing the diaphragm to spasm. Any coarse substance, such as salt, will have the same effect—but sugar tastes better!

3 DARK CHOCOLATE

Researchers have found that the theobromine in dark chocolate is more effective than codeine at suppressing a persistent cough without side effects such as drowsiness and constipation.

4 HONEY

To calm a nagging cough that keeps you awake at night, take 2 teaspoons of honey along with 500 milligrams of Ester C 30 minutes before bed. Recent studies have shown that honey works better than either a cough suppressant or no treatment at all for relieving nocturnal cough and promoting sleep. The vitamin C helps boosts the immune system in the early stages of your cough. (Note: Honey should not be given to children under age 1.)

5 LINDEN FLOWER

A tea made from this herb helps to cool a fever in two ways: It stimulates the hypothalamus to better regulate your temperature; and it dilates blood vessels, inducing sweating. Steep 1 tablespoon of the dried herb (available in health food stores) in a cup of hot water for 15 minutes, then allow to cool. Drink three to four cups a day. If you still run hot after a day of sipping tea, seek medical attention.

6 PEPPERMINT

Peppermint kills the bacteria that cause bloating and relaxes gastrointestinal muscles for smoother, spasm-free digestion. To quiet flatulence, take two enteric-coated peppermint capsules (500 milligrams each) three times daily. The enteric coating prevents the capsules from opening in the stomach, where they could increase discomfort by causing heartburn and indigestion. Instead, the peppermint releases and goes to work lower in the gastrointestinal tract, where gas-plagued people need it most.

7 CHERRIES

To encourage a good night's sleep, eat at a handful of cherries before bedtime. Scientists have discovered that the luscious red fruit is jam-packed with melatonin, the same hormone produced by your body to regulate sleep patterns.

8 STRAWBERRIES

The astringent malic acid in strawberries helps buff coffee and red-wine stains from teeth. Crush a few fresh strawberries into a scrubbing pulp, then mix with a pinch of stain-removing baking soda and enough water to make a paste. Apply this mixture to a soft-bristled toothbrush and polish for a few minutes once every 3 or 4 months. (More often than that could erode tooth enamel.)

9 OATS

Although oatmeal is a centuries-old skin soother, researchers only recently discovered that the avenanthramides in oats are responsible for calming inflamed,

itchy skin. Put whole oats in a clean, dry sock. Seal the open end with a rubber band and drop the sock into a warm or hot bath. Climb in and soak for 15 to 20 minutes.

10 BLACK TEA

If a late night at the office leaves you with puffy, tired eyes, revive them with chilled black tea bags. Black tea is chock-full of tannins, astringent compounds that can help deflate and tighten the bags under your eyes. Activate the tannins by dipping two tea bags in a cup of hot water for several minutes. Cool in the fridge, then apply the damp bags as a compress to closed eyes for 10 minutes.

your list

7 questions to ask your doctor

mini LIST

Stop MRSA

Methicillin-resistant *Staphylococcus aureus* (MRSA) is a drug-resistant bacteria commonly found in hospitals. Ask these questions to reduce your chances of infection:

1. **What is your infection rate?** "Hospitals may not thoroughly monitor all kinds of infection. But it doesn't hurt to ask," says Christine Nutty, RN, MSN, CIC, president of the Association for Professionals in Infection Control and Epidemiology.

2. **Have you washed your hands?** If the doctor hesitates, ask him or her to scrub up.

3. **Will you use a razor?** Razor blades can cause microscopic nicks that open the skin to infection. Nutty recommends asking the nurse or surgeon to use clippers with a disposable blade.

KEEPING AN OPEN line of communication between patient and health-care professional is more important than ever, especially now, as more people are researching health information on the Internet. Knowing which questions to ask your doctor can seem daunting, so follow this script from the National Institutes of Health to get started.

1 IS THIS TEST REALLY NECESSARY?

Before having a medical test, ask your doctor to explain why it is important, what it will show, and what it will cost. Also ask what you need to do to prepare for the test. For example, you may need to fast beforehand or provide a urine sample. Ask how you will be notified of the test results and how long they will take to come in.

2 WHAT MAY HAVE CAUSED THIS CONDITION?

When the test results are back, discuss your diagnosis and what you can expect. Will the condition be permanent? What will be the long-term effects on your life? Also ask if you should watch for any particular symptoms and notify your physician when they occur. Finally, ask if you should make any lifestyle changes due to your new diagnosis.

3 WHAT ARE MY TREATMENT OPTIONS?

Ask about the treatment for your condition, when it can start, and how long it will last. You should leave the doctor's office knowing both the benefits and risks of the treatment, and the overall success rate. Ask if there are any foods, drinks, or activities you should avoid while being treated.

4 COULD MEDICINE HELP?

If your doctor prescribes a drug for your condition, ask about the common side effects, and when the medicine should begin to work. As with other types of treatment, ask if there are foods, drinks, or activities you should avoid while you are taking the medicine. If you are taking other medications, make sure your doctor knows so he or she can prevent harmful drug interactions.

5 ARE THERE ANY OTHER SIDE EFFECTS?

Sometimes medicines affect people differently, so let the doctor know if your medicine doesn't seem to be working or if it is causing problems. Some side effects happen just when you start taking the medicine. Some happen once in a while and you learn how to manage them. It is best not to stop taking the medicine on your own. If you want to stop taking your medicine, always consult your doctor first.

6 WHAT IS YOUR SUCCESS RATE?

If you need surgery, ask not only the success rate of the operation, but how many of these the surgeon has done successfully. Also find out if you must be admitted to a hospital, or if it could be an outpatient procedure.

When surgery is recommended, many people often seek a second opinion. In fact, many insurance plans today require it. Doctors are used to this practice, and most will not be offended by your request for a second opinion. Your doctor may even be able to suggest other doctors who can review your case.

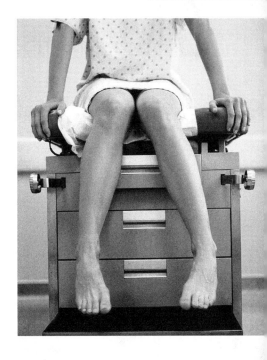

7 WHEN DO YOU MAKE ROUNDS?

If you have to be hospitalized, remember that doctors generally make rounds at about the same time every day. Ask when the doctor is likely to visit your room so you can have questions ready.

your list

6 tips for a good night's sleep

facts & figures

54°
to 75°F

The ideal room temperature for a good night's sleep, according to the National Sleep Foundation.

WE ARE A nation plagued by sleeplessness. According to the National Institutes of Health, 50 to 70 million Americans are affected by chronic sleep disorders and intermittent sleep problems that can negatively impact health, alertness, and safety. Untreated sleep disorders have been linked to hypertension, heart disease, stroke, diabetes, and depression, among other chronic conditions.

If you think getting a good night's sleep is someone else's dream, think again. Follow these tips, and you'll be snoozing in no time.

1 SKIP THE NIGHTCAP

Alcohol is probably the substance used most often for sleep, reports a study in *Principles and Practice of Sleep Medicine*. However, when you fall asleep under the influence, both the quantity and the quality of your sleep are adversely affected. Even small to moderate intakes of alcohol can suppress melatonin (a hormone that helps regulate sleep), interfere with restorative N-REM cycles, and prevent dreaming, according to Rubin Naiman, PhD, a clinical assistant professor of medicine at the Arizona Center for Integrative Medicine at the University of Arizona and coauthor of *Healthy Sleep*.

2 JUNK THE JAVA

Caffeine enhances alertness, activates stress hormones, and elevates heart rate and blood pressure—none of which is very helpful when you're trying to get shut-eye. If you are sensitive to caffeine, take note that its half-life—the time required for your body to break down half of it—can be as long as 7 hours. In women, estrogen may delay caffeine metabolism even more. In the days between ovulation and menstruation, it takes about 25% longer for a woman to eliminate caffeine; for women using birth control pills, elimination time can double. (Newer, low-estrogen pills may have less of an impact, however.)

Coffee, tea, chocolate, energy/sport drinks, and soft drinks all contain caffeine. It's also added to over-the-counter medications such as pain relievers, appetite suppressants, and cold medicines.

3 TURN DOWN THE HEAT

Most sleep researchers recommend keeping your bedroom cool but not cold. This allows your core body temperature to drop, which helps to induce sleep. The thermostat is only part of the story, however. Proper air circulation and lighter-weight blankets also can facilitate a drop in body temperature.

Swiss researchers Kurt Kräuchi and Anna Wirz-Justice, PhD, found an inverse relationship between warm extremities and cool body temperature. When your feet and hands are warm, your blood vessels dilate. This allows heat to escape and body temperature to fall, initiating sleep. Conversely, when your hands and feet are cold, your blood vessels constrict to retain heat—and you stay awake.

4 DON'T WORK OUT WITHIN 3 HOURS OF BEDTIME

Physical activity raises core body temperature, which is why we're advised to skip exercise in the evening. The issue isn't quite so cut-and-dried, however. Some studies show evening activity to be bad for sleep, while others have found a positive effect. According to Gayle Greene, author of *Insomniac*, "You need to find what works for you. I found that if I didn't exercise, I'd feel worse and my health would suffer, and that would ultimately undermine my sleep."

5 DEVELOP A SLEEP RITUAL

Experts suggest engaging in relaxing activities in the evening to prepare yourself for slumber. "It should be something that you do every night to signal to your body that it's time to unwind," explains Michael Breus, PhD, clinical director of the sleep division of Southwest Sport and Spine in Scottsdale, Arizona, and a clinical psychologist who's board-certified in clinical sleep disorders.

6 SET A REGULAR SLEEP-WAKE SCHEDULE

Most experts advise that we go to bed and wake up at the same time every day. They point to evidence that our circadian rhythms—the natural ebb and flow of energy levels that occurs throughout the day—thrive on consistency. The more predictable our sleep schedule, the better our bodies work, the theory goes.

But even those who most strongly espouse this view admit that while adhering to a regular sleep-wake schedule is helpful, it may not be the complete answer. "Even if insomniacs keep regular sleep patterns, it doesn't necessarily mean they'll sleep well or long enough," says Kathryn Reid, PhD, research assistant professor in the department of neurology at the North-western University Center for Sleep and Circadian Rhythm.

your list

7 ways to wake up your energy

facts & figures

18,000
to
20,000

The number of breaths you take each day. Boost your energy by practicing stress-busting techniques such as deep breathing as often as you can.

"YOUTH IS WASTED on the young," the saying goes. Indeed, as we look back on our teens and 20s, we wonder how we managed to stay out on the town until 2 o'clock in the morning and then wake up 4 hours later, refreshed and ready to go. If only we could recapture that energy and use it for more noble purposes, like not drifting off at our desks by mid-afternoon.

It is possible to recapture that youthful vim and vigor, to stay alert and "on" all day long. Start with this collection of natural energizers.

1 LIGHTEN UP

Instead of sleeping in, try getting up at your usual time and soaking in some natural light. This enables your circadian rhythms—which are governed by the "master clock" in your hypothalamus gland—to stay in sync with the 24-hour day. Aim for 30 minutes of light first thing in the morning, even on weekends. You can start your day by taking a half-hour stroll outdoors or by having your breakfast by a sunny window. If your schedule requires you to rise while it's dark outside, flip on the lights indoors. Every little bit of light may help!

2 BE PRUDENT WITH CARBS

Although they're a ready energy source, carbohydrates can be an energy drain if they're eaten in excess. Women who reduced the carbs in their diets while increasing protein felt more energetic, according to a study by Donald K. Layman, PhD, professor of nutrition at the University of Illinois. Keep your daily intake of healthy complex carbs below 150 grams, best apportioned as follows: five servings of vegetables; two servings of fruit; and three or four servings of starchy (preferably whole grain) carbohydrates such as breads, rice, pastas, and cereals.

3 TAKE AN AFTERNOON COFFEE BREAK

Instead of downing your cuppa first thing in the morning, save it for later in the day. Caffeine blocks the effects of adenosine, a sleep-inducing brain chemical that accumulates as the day wears on. By the time adenosine builds up to the point where you start feeling sleepy—generally, in late afternoon—the effects of your morning caffeine will have worn off, says James K. Wyatt, PhD, director of the Sleep Disorders Service and Research Center at Rush University Medical Center. Note: If you're highly sensitive to caffeine's effects, plan your coffee break for early afternoon, so you don't have difficulty falling asleep at night.

4 SQUEEZE IN STRESS-BUSTERS

"Even in the span of 3 minutes, meditation can reduce the stress hormones that tense your muscles and constrict your blood vessels," says Judith Orloff, MD, a psychiatrist at UCLA and author of *Positive Energy*. "It increases endorphins, too." To practice meditation, find a quiet place where you won't be interrupted. Sit down and close your eyes. Focus on your breath as you slowly inhale and exhale; as thoughts intrude, imagine that they're clouds floating by in the sky. Then visualize something or someone who makes you happy.

5 BEAT AN AFTERNOON SLUMP

Instead of hunkering down for a power nap, take a walk outdoors. Just as it does in the early morning, light later in the day may blunt an afternoon energy dip, which often comes on like clockwork. "Because of the way in which homeostatic and circadian systems interact, most people feel a lull 17 to 18 hours after they went to bed the previous night," notes Mariana Figueiro, PhD, program director of the Lighting Research Center at Rensselaer Polytechnic Institute.

6 GET PUMPED BEFORE A WORKOUT

Exercise is among the most effective energizers around. But what if you're too tired for a good workout? Put in your

earphones while you lace up your walking shoes: Music will help you forget you're whipped. Volunteers who exercised for 30 minutes while listening to tunes felt as though they weren't exerting themselves as much as when they worked out without music, Japanese researchers reported in the *Journal of Sports Medicine and Physical Fitness*. So load your iPod or mix CD with your favorite up-tempo tunes and get moving!

7 UNWIND BEFORE BED

"Studies show that very bright light—the equivalent to early morning outdoor light—increases brain activity," Figueiro says. Some scientists believe that even the light emitted by a computer monitor late at night can confuse your body's sleep-wake cycle. Wind down by watching TV instead. Most people sit far enough away from the television (at least 15 feet) to be unaffected by its brightness. Better yet, read a book or magazine. Just make sure that your reading light doesn't exceed 60 watts. And log off your computer at least an hour before bedtime.

your list

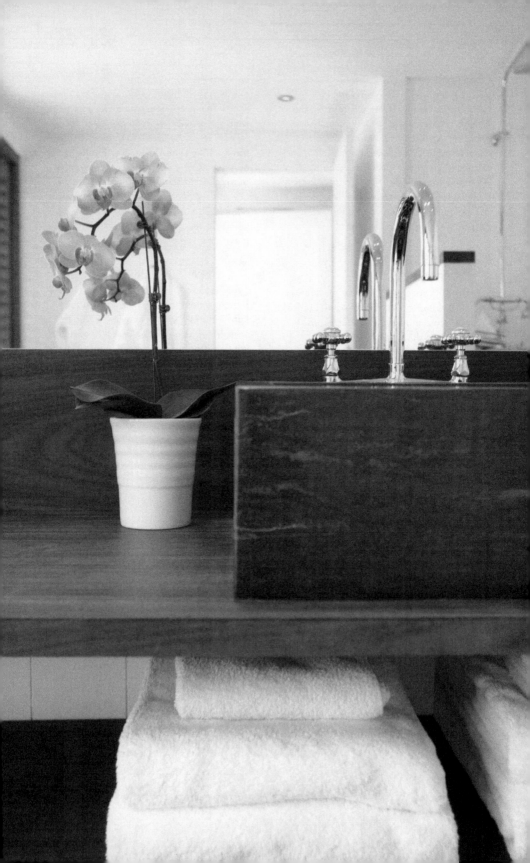

chapter 6 # home

top 10 easy ways to be "green"

mini LIST

How to smoke out leaks

Finding air leaks in your home isn't difficult. All you need is a little detective work—and an incense stick! Here's how to ID energy bandits and put the air in your home on lockdown. (Note: This works best on a cool, windy day, when drafts are most noticeable.)

1. Turn off your furnace.

2. Close all of your windows and doors.

3. Turn on any exhaust fans that vent outside, like kitchen and bathroom fans.

4. Light an incense stick and pass it around common air leak sites like window and door frames, vents, air conditioners, and cable and phone lines. If smoke is sucked out of or blown into the room, you've found a leak.

TODAY, APPROXIMATELY 10% of homes under construction in the United States are considered green, compared with just 2% in 2005. They are built from toxin-free materials and have energy-efficient features that not only are environmentally friendly but save homeowners money in the long run. Green homes use 40% less energy than standard homes, according to the United States Green Building Council (USGBC).

But what if you aren't in the market for a new home? No matter where you live, there's much you can do to create a healthier living space, be kind to the environment, and cut your energy costs. For example:

1 WASH FULL LOADS
You'll save at least 3,400 gallons of water a year if you wash only full loads of laundry, according to the USGBC.

2 TRY COLD WATER
About 90% of the energy used to wash clothes goes toward heating the water. Wash your clothes in cold water using a cold-water detergent whenever possible. You'll not only save money by not heating the water, you'll also lessen CO_2 emissions. Just think: If everyone in the United States washed their clothes in cold water, it would reduce our nation's CO_2 emissions by 47 million tons per year!

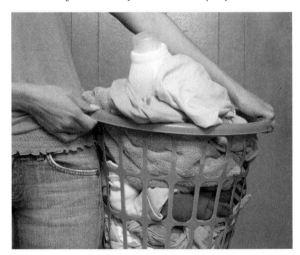

3 USE CFLs

By replacing five of your most frequently used incandescent light bulbs with compact fluorescent light bulbs (CFLs), you'll save over $100 a year. If every family in the United States did this, greenhouse gas emissions would decline by 1 trillion pounds.

4 FLIP THE SWITCH

For lights with incandescent bulbs, turn them off when they aren't in use. Only 5 to 15% of the energy drawn by incandescent bulbs is used for light. The rest is just waste heat, says Harvey M. Sachs, PhD, senior fellow of the American Council for an Energy Efficient Economy's Building Program, based in Washington, DC.

5 PROGRAM THERMOSTATS

Turn down thermostats when you aren't at home or you're sleeping, and you'll save 10% on heating and cooling costs. What are the most efficient settings for summer and winter? The settings closest to the outdoor temperature that you can tolerate, Sachs says.

6 STOP AIR LEAKS

They are the biggest energy drain, and they also happen to be easiest to fix. Weatherstripping and/or caulking will do the trick.

7 WIPE YOUR FEET!

According to the Washington Toxics Coalition, using entryway mats can reduce the amount of toxic residues on carpets by 25% and dust on carpets by 33%. Homes where shoes are left at the door have 10 times less dust than homes where shoes are worn inside.

8 CHOOSE ENERGY STAR

Americans using Energy Star appliances, lights, and windows saved $12 billion in 2005, and enough energy to equal the emissions from 23 million cars.

9 BUY A PLANT

Paints, varnishes, cleaning supplies, computer printers, and even air fresheners release pollutants called volatile organic compounds, or VOCs. Australian researchers have discovered that houseplants, specifically Janet Crain and Sweet Chico, reduce VOCs by up to 70%. Plants pull in pollutants floating in the air. The toxins travel to the roots, where soil breaks them down into nontoxic compounds that the plant then uses for food.

10 UNPLUG

When electronics are turned off, they are in "standby" mode, which means they're continuing to use energy. Almost any device in your home that has a remote control, continuous LED display, soft touch keypad, or external power source or that charges batteries is drawing standby energy. According to the US Department of Energy, 75% of the electricity that powers appliances and electronics is used while they are turned off. In an average home, at least 20 devices use standby energy. So when you aren't using electronics such as computers, printers, and AC adaptors, unplug them.

your list

10 tips to keep appliances in shape

my favorite...
Way to Clean
a Stove Vent Filter

Teresa Hunsaker, family
and consumer science
educator

"A dirty stove vent filter
not only compromises
the performance of your
stove, it also could be a
fire hazard," Hunsaker
says. Her tip for cleaning
a filter: Soak it in good
old ammonia and water.
"Let it sit for 30 to 40
minutes in 5 parts hot
water to 1 part ammo-
nia," she recommends.
"Then gently scrub it
with a brush and rinse it
with water, and you're
good to go."

WE'VE BEEN USING essentially the same array of appliances for decades, but the 21st-century models are designed to lessen their environmental impact, save energy, and lighten our utility bills. Refrigerators and freezers of today, for instance, are three times more efficient than those of 30 years ago. They have more insulation, better door seals, and advanced temperature controls. Replace a 1980s fridge with one of today's innovative versions, and you'll save more than $100 in utility bills every year.

Regardless of make and model, all appliances need to be maintained properly to operate at peak efficiency. Clogged vents, greasy burners, and encrusted filters force them to work harder and use more energy. Older appliances, in particular, can be energy hogs if they aren't maintained properly. They also can operate just as efficiently as new models when given a little TLC. Here's how to make the most of your energy dollars and prevent your appliances from blowing a gasket.

1 STICK TO SCHEDULES

If your home has a forced air heating and cooling system, as most American homes do, the air filter should be replaced or cleaned according to schedule. This means every 1 to 2 months for common "rock catcher" air filters. For 4-inch-deep pleated filters, annual replacement is sufficient, says Harvey M. Sachs, PhD. Electrostatic or electronic filters have their own schedules; some can be cleaned in the dishwasher.

2 GIVE YOUR AC SOME SPACE

An outdoor central air conditioning unit needs to "breathe." Keep surrounding foliage trimmed back, and don't surround the unit with fencing, which will block air flow. In general, manufacturers recommend an annual or bi-annual "tune-up" for the system, but oil-fired equipment requires annual service, Sachs says.

In the fall, cover your AC to prevent dust and debris from collecting around it.

3 REPLACE SCREENS

According to the U.S. Department of Energy, you should replace window and door screens with storm windows when the temperatures begin to drop. They provide an extra barrier against cold temperatures and winter winds.

4 DEFROST YOUR FRIDGE

Refrigerators with auto-defrost use more energy than models that are manual defrost, but the manual kind can be just as wasteful. The reason: Any amount of frost buildup reduces the efficiency of the freezer. Once frost accumulates to more than ¼ inch thick, it's time for a cleaning.

5 CHECK THE SEAL

Periodically check the refrigerator gasket to make sure that caked-on food isn't stopping the door from sealing tightly.

6 CLEAR THE AIRWAY

Clean your dryer vent duct at least once a year to prevent heat buildup. Also inspect your dryer vent periodically to make sure that it's not blocked. This simple step not only saves energy, it also could prevent a fire.

7 GIVE LINT THE BRUSH-OFF

Clean the dryer lint filter or trap before every load. A clogged filter keeps moist air from escaping, so the dryer has to work longer and harder to do its job. Clearing the lint before each load will save you up to $34 a year.

8 LET THERE BE LIGHT

Wipe dust and dirt from lamps and lighting fixtures every 6 to 24 months. Accumulating dust reduces illumination by 50% or more, but your lights will continue to use full power. Turn your lights off while cleaning, especially when wiping an incandescent light bulb. Cool moisture can cause the hot bulb to shatter.

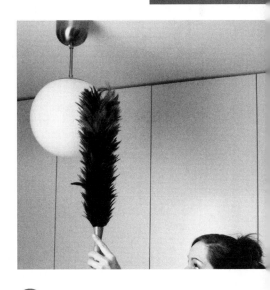

9 DON'T LET DUST SETTLE

Dust on the surfaces that surround your lighting fixtures limits the amount of reflected light, says the US Department of Energy. Keep these surfaces clean and free of debris.

10 DE-GRIME THE STOVE

When blackened with cooking spills and grease, the plates under conventional coil burners don't reflect heat well. They should be shiny so that they absorb the maximum amount of heat. Also, don't forget to clean the stove vent filter every six months, advises Teresa Hunsaker, family and consumer science educator at Utah State University Extension in Logan. An accumulation of grease will stop heat and odors from escaping.

your list
_____

_____

_____

_____

_____

_____

5 green cleaning-product swaps

facts & figures

240
thousand

The number of jobs generated by the manufacturing of green products in 2007. Green services, ranging from energy conservation to pollution control, accounted for 1.4 million to 1.8 million jobs. According to a 2010 report by the Economics and Statistics Administration of the US Department of Commerce, the development of the green industry is a rising contributor to economic growth.

A CLEAN APPLIANCE is an efficient appliance. Without dirt and grime to gum up the works, appliances purr at maximum efficiency. But before you scrub and buff, take a look at the cleaners you're using. Most of them have their own environmental effects.

You can take your greening efforts a step farther by stocking up on cleaning products that are toxin-free. "They pose fewer dangers but retain their ability to dissolve stains, fats, and oils," notes Howard Hu, MD, PhD, ScD, chair of the Department of Environmental Health Sciences at the University of Michigan Schools of Public Health in Ann Arbor.

This list homes in on five product categories that commonly use hazardous ingredients in their formulas. It also includes alternative eco-friendly products you can find in most stores. (For more product recommendations, visit www.epa.gov/dfe and www.greenseal.org.)

1 DISHWASHING DETERGENTS

The chemicals in hand dishwashing detergents tend to be milder than those in dishwasher detergents. However, they still contain ingredients to be wary of. Many are heavy in inorganic phosphates, chemicals that diminish oxygen levels in the water and harm aquatic life. Any ingredient accompanied by the word "cationic," "anionic," or "nonionic" contain phosphates.

Cleaner Alternatives:
- Green Works Natural Dishwashing Liquid—Free & Clear, Original, Simply Lemon, Tangerine, Water Lily (The Clorox Company)
- Palmolive Ultra Original Dishwashing Liquid (Colgate-Palmolive Company)
- Hand Dish Liquid—Free & Clear, Lavender Floral, Lemongrass (Seventh Generation)

2 ALL-PURPOSE CLEANERS

These can contain any number of toxic chemicals to disinfect and cut grease—and to smell nice while doing it.

Ingredients like ammonia, ethelyne glycol, and monobuytl acetate disturb the delicate pH balance of fresh water. And the sweet smells can induce wildlife to drink the hazardous solutions.

Cleaner Alternatives:

- Earth Choice All Purpose Cleaner and Degreaser (Clean Control Corporation)
- Green All Purpose Cleaner (Crescent Manufacturing)
- Legacy of Clean Concentrated Multi-Purpose Cleaner (Amway Global)
- Office Depot Green All Purpose Cleaner (Office Depot)
- Sustainable Earth by Staples Multi-Purpose Cleaner (Staples Contract & Commercial, Inc.)

3 WINDOW AND GLASS CLEANERS

They commonly contain isopropanol—an ingredient that's harmful to aquatic life—and ammonia. Toxicology research shows that isopropanol alcohol affects the stages of growth in animals.

Cleaner Alternatives:

- Earth Choice Glass & Surface Cleaner (Clean Control Corporation)
- Green Works Natural Glass and Surface Cleaner—Original (The Clorox Company)
- Window Kleener with Lavender and Window Kleener with Vinegar (Earth Friendly Products)
- Blue Window Glass Cleaner (Berkley Packaging Company)

4 FURNITURE POLISHES AND CLEANERS

Wood polishes and oils may contain petroleum distillates and volatile oils that actually attract dust. Always use polishes in ventilated areas.

Cleaner Alternatives:

- Green World Furniture Cleaner and Polish (Chase Products Company)
- GreenLight Wood & All Surface 201 Cleaner (MainTex, Inc.)

5 RUG AND CARPET CLEANERS

The main ingredients in these products are perchloroethylene, or perc, and naphthalene. Perc is a solvent commonly used by dry cleaners. Naphthalene has the distinct odor of mothballs; it evaporates quickly and has damaging effects in the atmosphere. When naphthalene is absorbed into the soil, it remains unchanged for many years.

Cleaner Alternatives:

- Carpet Spot and Stain Remover (HAZfree, Inc.)
- Perfect Planet Carpet Cleaner (Weiman Products LLC)
- Simple Green Naturals Floor Care (Simple Green)
- Responsibly Clean Rug and Carpet Cleaner (Nexgen Chemistries)

your list

11 DIY "green" cleaning products

Sarah Hodgson, author of *Puppies for Dummies*

Lifting pet stains off carpet is not just a cosmetic challenge; animal excrement is full of bacteria and possibly parasites. "The most important thing to do is break up the enzymes in the urine or stool," Hodgson advises. "The enzymes are what encourage your pet to mark that spot again and again." Hodgson's recipe: Fill a spray bottle with a half-and-half mixture of apple cider or white vinegar and water. Saturate the area with solution and pat dry with a paper towel. Repeat, then let dry.

MANY RECIPES FOR homemade cleaning products have survived for generations. And for good reason: They work, they're safe, and they're less expensive than store-bought cleaners. If you want to avoid the hydroxides, the chlorides, and the peroxides and use a gentler means to clean, try these green solutions.

1 RUG AND CARPET STAIN REMOVER
To remove stains, add ½ cup of vinegar and 2 to 3 tablespoons of baking soda to 4 cups of warm water. Stir slightly and allow to fizz and foam. Then dip a brush in the mixture and scrub the stain, advises Teresa Hunsaker, family and consumer science educator. Vacuum the rug or carpet when it's dry.

2 GLASS CLEANER
Many glass cleaners contain ammonia, a known toxin. A safer option suggested by the Environmental Protection Agency is vinegar. Add ¼ to ½ cup of white vinegar to a quart of warm water. Pour the solution into a spray bottle and use as needed. Rub dry with newspaper, which doesn't leave lint behind and coats glass with a dirt-resistant film.

3 BATHTUB STAIN REMOVER
For tub stains, fill a small shallow bowl with cream of tartar. Add drops of hydrogen peroxide until a thick paste forms. Apply to the stain and let dry. When the paste is rinsed away, the stain is gone.

4 MOLD AND MILDEW LIFTER
Mold and mildew on bathroom fixtures can be especially stubborn. Make a paste of baking soda and cool water. Spread it over the entire surface and allow to sit for a few minutes. Rinse with cold water.

5 SHOWERHEAD CLEANER
Remove the showerhead and soak in a solution of 2 cups white vinegar and 2 cups warm water. Let it set for

several hours or overnight. Then rinse the head with water to remove deposits. If some deposits remain, Hunsaker says, gently scrub them with a scrubbing pad or cloth.

For a non-removable showerhead, soak a towel in the vinegar-water solution and wrap it around the head. Tie a plastic bag around the towel to help retain moisture. Remove it after several hours and wipe away the deposits.

6 FAUCET BRIGHTENER

Dingy faucets can be restored to their shiny former selves. Dissolve 4 tablespoons of table salt in ¼ cup of vinegar. Dip a sponge or soft cloth in the solution and wipe down the faucet and handles. Then rinse thoroughly and polish dry with a clean cloth.

7 OVEN CLEANER

A self-cleaning oven heats up to 900°F to incinerate food particles and spills. No matter how tightly sealed the oven is, it will release smoke, fumes, and carbon monoxide. A more eco-friendly alternative: Sprinkle baking soda in a ¼-inch layer and spritz with water until it's damp, says Annie Bond, author of *Better Basics for the Home: Simple Solutions for Less Toxic Living*. Let it set overnight; the grime should lift right off the next day.

8 KITCHEN COUNTER DE-STAINER

For a Formica countertop that's stained, Hunsaker recommends the one-two punch of lemon juice and baking soda. First squeeze a fresh lemon over the stain and let it soak for 30 minutes. Next, sprinkle baking soda over the juice. Scrub with a terrycloth rag, rinse, and wipe dry.

9 CLOG DISSOLVER

For greasy clogged drains, pour ½ cup of salt, ½ cup of vinegar, and ½ cup of baking soda down the drain. Immediately follow with at least 2 quarts of boiling water as a chaser, Hunsaker says.

10 GARBAGE DISPOSAL DEODORIZER

Freeze ½ cup of lemon juice or vinegar in an ice cup tray. Grind the cubes in the disposal once a week. The ice cubes sharpen the blades, while the lemon juice or vinegar keeps the disposal smelling fresh.

11 DISHWASHER DETERGENT

Forgo the commercial dishwasher detergents, with their hazardous chlorine and surfactants, and use two common household ingredients instead. Fill the soap dispenser with a mix of one part borax and one part baking soda. Borax has safe bleaching and stain-removing properties.

your list

_____

_____

_____

_____

_____

_____

_____

_____

_____

_____

7 tips to store food safely

facts & figures

76
million

The number of Americans who experience foodborne illnesses each year, according to the Centers for Disease Control and Prevention. Among the most vulnerable are childern, the elderly, and those with weakened immune systems.

GENERALLY, SPOILAGE ISN'T hard to spot. Mold, unpleasant odors, and slimy textures are dead giveaways. But "you can't always count on sight or smell to tell you whether food is good to eat," says Elizabeth L. Andress, PhD, a food safety specialist at the University of Georgia. The expiration date on the product packaging is the most reliable indicator of a food's status. And of course, always remember to heed the words of food safety experts: When in doubt, throw it out!

There are some simple things that can be done to preserve a food's freshness and keep spoilage at bay for a while longer. The secret to extending shelf life is to keep out air and moisture, says Teresa Hunsaker, family and consumer science educator. Here's what she and other experts recommend.

1 TAKE THE TEMPERATURE

For foods to remain their freshest, your refrigerator should be set at 40°F or lower. Higher temperatures will speed up spoilage. Keep in mind, though, that just storing food at the proper temperature isn't enough to stop spoilage. "Many people don't understand that while refrigeration slows bacterial growth, it doesn't stop completely," says Janet B. Anderson, RD, clinical professor of nutrition and food sciences at Utah State University. In one study, Anderson and her research team found that 31% of respondents ate refrigerated leftovers that were over a week old, long enough for mold to grow and food to spoil.

2 POSTPONE PURCHASING PERISHABLES

When doing your grocery shopping, save the meat, poultry, and eggs for last, so they stay refrigerated longer, the US Department of Agriculture recommends. Also, once you've made your purchases, try to get them home and into your refrigerator within 2 hours—1 hour if the outside temperature is 90°F or higher.

3 BROWN-BAG MUSHROOMS

"Mushrooms contain a lot of moisture, so they grow icky fast," Hunsaker says. Remove them from their container and put them in a paper bag. Fold over the top edge of the bag, secure it with a clip, and put the bag in your crisper drawer.

4 SET A DATE

To keep track of when you opened an item or put leftovers in the fridge, mark the date on masking tape and attach it to the package or container.

5 KEEP FRESH-BAKED COOKIES FRESH

After the cookies have cooled, put them in an air-tight container or a zip-top bag along with a slice of bread. The starch in the bread absorbs moisture, so the cookies stay soft and fresh. When the bread goes stale, replace with a new slice to help your cookies last longer.

6 MAKE CHEESE LAST

Dip a cheese cloth in undiluted white vinegar and wring it out. Wrap the cloth around your brick of cheese. Then wrap the cheese in aluminum foil and put it in an airtight plastic storage bag. The vinegar inhibits mold growth, extending the shelf life of the cheese by 3 to 6 weeks. "Not to worry—you won't taste the vinegar," Hunsaker says.

7 PUT BREAD ON ICE

Many people store their bread in the refrigerator. While the cold temperature will slow mold growth, it also dries out the bread. Instead, Hunsaker recommends storing the bread in the freezer as individual slices and thawing them as you need them. Or double-bag the bread, leaving as little trapped air in the bag as possible. If your bread turns stale, simply put it on a cookie sheet, sprinkle it with a little water, and pop it into a 350°F oven for a few minutes.

your list

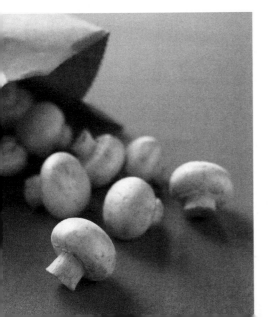

5 essential tests for your home

mini LIST

Get the lead out

If your water contains lead, flush it out with these tips:

- Run your tap for 15 to 20 seconds to eliminate water that's been sitting in the pipes for a few hours.

- Cook with cold water.

- Consider buying a water filter approved by NSF International or the Water Quality Association.

NOT EVERYTHING NATURAL is good for you. Radon, for example, is a byproduct of decay in the soil, and mold is a fungus in search of some moisture and a surface to settle on and grow.

Then there are the man-made pollutants like carbon monoxide (CO) and lead. You may not be able to see, smell, or taste them, but with the right tools, you can detect them.

In fact, our experts recommend home tests for all four of these substances, plus your water quality. The tests can give you peace of mind—or allow you to take action before a problem gets out of hand. Here's what you need to know.

1 RADON

Radon is the second leading cause of lung cancer, right behind smoking. Fortunately, radon testing is simple and inexpensive. Choose either a short-term test kit, which measures radioactive concentrations for up to several months, or a long-term kit that monitors continuously for a year. The World Health Organization recommends the long-term kits for a more accurate assessment, since radon concentrations can fluctuate significantly over time.

If you use a short-term kit and you get a reading of 4 pCi/L or higher, the Environmental Protection Agency suggests following up with a second short-term test. If the average of the two tests is 4 pCi/L, then consider taking steps to reduce the radon level in your home. Contact your state's radon office to find a contractor, or visit the EPA website (www.epa.gov) for information on correcting the problem yourself.

2 CARBON MONOXIDE

Carbon monoxide (CO) poisoning is an especially common home health hazard during the winter months. That's when fuel-burning appliances such as fireplaces, wood stoves, and heaters can pollute indoor air if they aren't maintained or functioning properly.

"To stay safe from CO poisoning, have all fuel-burning appliances inspected and cleaned by a professional, and install at least one CO detector to alert you to dangerous levels of the deadly gas in your home," says Meri-K Appy, president of the Home Safety Council in Washington, DC. Choose a detector that has been tested by a recognized laboratory (look for ETL, UL, or CSA on the label) and mount it near the sleeping areas of your home.

3 WATER

If your community's water supply serves more than 100,000 people, you can access a water quality report at www.epa.gov. Once you've read the report, you may decide to have your home's water evaluated. In that case, your state certification officer can recommend a certified laboratory. You can locate and contact your state certification officer by searching the EPA Web site or by calling EPA's Safe Drinking Water Hotline at (800) 426-4791. Be aware that water quality tests can range in price from $15 to hundreds of dollars.

If you live in one of the 50 million US households that rely on private wells, check yours annually to make sure that the water is safe to drink. Testing by a certified laboratory can cost anywhere from $10 to several thousand dollars, depending on the number of chemicals assessed.

4 MOLD

You'll never escape mold spores and mold, but you can control overgrowth by limiting moisture. You can find out if overgrowth is a problem simply by looking for it. Check bathrooms, refrigerators, attics, basements, and other areas that tend to collect moisture. Condensation on the inside of windows, walls, and pipes are signs that your home is humid and likely to breed mold. Use dehumidifiers, ventilators, air conditioners, and exhaust fans to reduce humidity.

If you do spot moisture, clean and dry the affected area as soon as possible. You can stop mold growth by drying the area within 24 to 48 hours. Sometimes mold can

lurk in less obvious places—behind drywall, under carpet, on top of ceiling tiles, and inside the roof. If your home smells musty but you can't find mold, or if mold covers more than 10 square feet, call a contractor with mold remediation experience.

5 LEAD

If your home was built prior to 1978, it could have metal-laced dust from deteriorating paint. If you're concerned about peeling or flaking lead paint, contact your state housing department for testing and lab recommendations or call The National Lead Information Center at (800) 424-LEAD.

Since 1986, lead has been banned from use in the manufacture of plumbing materials. The same law allows manufacturers to label products as "lead-free" if they contain 8% or less lead. So any home—no matter when it was built—could have lead in its plumbing, including faucets that contain brass, says Veronica Blette, special assistant to the director of the EPA Office of Ground Water and Drinking Water. If you are concerned about lead, contact your local water authority to see if your home can be evaluated for free. Home testing kits also are available.

your list

12 ways to allergy-proof your home

mini LIST

Surprising places where allergens lurk

Pollen may not be the reason for the sneezin'. There are plenty of other culprits (dander, mold, dust) lurking around your home. Here are some of their hideouts:

- Guests with pets may unwittingly drag pet allergens into your home. Vacuum the upholstery after they've left.

- Books and other shelf-dwellers contribute dust and mold. Dust and wipe down books and trinkets at least once a week.

- Refrigerator gaskets collect spills and crumbs, making them a breeding ground for mold. Wipe the seal with bleach and water weekly.

- Moist bath mats allow dust mites and mold to thrive. After a shower, hang up the mat and run the fan or open a window.

ACCORDING TO THE American Academy of Allergy, Asthma, and Immunology, millions of Americans are allergic to certain substances that populate indoor air. These allergens continuously parade around every home, challenging immune systems and inducing noses to run, eyes to water, and skin to itch. Fortunately, you can get the upper hand on airborne irritants with a little bit of vigilance and simple tactics like these.

1 PUT DUST MITES TO REST

The most common triggers of allergy and asthma symptoms are the droppings left by dust mites, which love to inhabit mattresses, pillows, bedding, and carpet. To keep these malevolent microbes at bay, encase mattresses, box springs, and pillows in allergen-free fabric or air-tight plastic covers. Wash bed linens in hot water (130°F) every week to kill dust mites and the allergens they leave behind. If you aren't able to wash comforters and pillows regularly, then cover them in allergen-free fabric as well.

2 VACUUM A LEAST ONCE A WEEK

This simple strategy lifts dust and dander from rugs and carpets. Consider purchasing a vacuum cleaner with a HEPA air filter or double up your vacuum bag.

3 CHOOSE CLOTHES MADE FROM NATURAL FIBERS

When synthetic fabrics rub against one another, they create an electrical charge that attracts pollen—which, as it turns out, has its own electrical charge, says Gailen D. Marshall, MD, PhD, director of clinical immunology and the Division of Allergy at the University of Mississippi. Natural fibers such as cotton also breathe better, so they stay drier and are less hospitable to moisture-loving mold.

4 DON'T HANG LAUNDRY ON CLOTHESLINES

Drying your clothes on an outdoor clothesline is eco-friendly, but if you're allergic to pollen, it's best to forgo this strategy. Pollen lands on your laundry, and then you carry it into your home—a formula for indoor contamination. Toss wet laundry in the dryer instead.

5 SHOWER IN THE EVENING

Bathing before bedtime will remove the dust and pollen that has collected on you and your clothing throughout the day, keeping your bed linens pollen-free.

6 REPLACE CARPETS WITH THROW RUGS

In rooms that are humid or tend to collect moisture, carpets can become a safe haven for mold. Throw rugs are a better choice because they can be washed and dried thoroughly on a regular basis. Your best bet, if you have a pollen or dust allergy: Replace wall-to-wall with linoleum or wood flooring, suggests the Academy of Family Physicians. Polished surfaces are easier to clean.

7 FIND A NEW HOME FOR HOUSEPLANTS

If you're sensitive to mold, send your houseplants packing. The soil is a breeding ground for mold, experts at the Mayo Clinic say. If you opt for artificial instead, be sure to wipe it down regularly. Artificial plants are dust magnets, as are knick-knacks, magazines, and newspapers.

8 DON'T LET PETS PEEVE YOU

Keep four-legged fluff balls out of your bedroom and any other room that you spend a lot of time in, Marshall says.

9 GROOM REGULARLY

Cats and dogs should be washed weekly and groomed several times a week. A bath and a brush remove loose hair, dust, pollen, and other allergy-inducing irritants.

10 RETHINK THE LITTER BOX

If you have a cat, assign litter box duty to someone else and place the box far away from any heating and air conditioning vents. If you must do clean-up yourself, wear a microfiber surgical mask, available at hardware and garden supply stores.

11 TOSS SCENTED CANDLES AND AIR FRESHENERS

"You're just masking a foul odor with a stronger odor," says James Sublett, MD, chief of pediatric allergy and immunology at the University of Louisville School of Medicine. Worse, candles give off soot particles, while candles and air fresheners give off synthetic fragrances—all of which trigger asthma and allergy symptoms. The healthiest way to eliminate odors in your home is to crack a window and turn on an exhaust fan. If you love the look of candles, try the unscented beeswax variety; they produce less soot and have a light honey fragrance that won't aggravate your symptoms.

12 BATTLE BUGS

Cockroach droppings have a protein that can trigger asthma symptoms in some people. Vacuum or sweep the floor after every meal, store food in airtight containers, remove garbage frequently, and adopt other clean practices that put out the "no vacancy" sign for roaming roaches.

your list

8 ways to accident-proof your home

facts & figures

83
percent

The number of parents who admit that they've left their toddlers without supervision for at least a few minutes, according to research by the Home Safety Council.

90
percent

The number of parents who say that their toddlers are up to something—climbing on furniture, tugging on curtains and tablecloths—as soon as their backs are turned.

EVEN AS GROWN-UPS, all of us have monsters in our closets—something that rattles our sense of safety, even in our own homes. For some it's thunderstorms; for others it's spiders and associated creepy-crawlies. But there are hazards around our homes that we ought to be much more wary of, in part because they're much more likely to harm us—seemingly innocuous things like high shelves, low lighting, and clutter. Consider this: On average, home injuries send some 21 million people to hospitals and doctors offices every year.

These types of injuries can happen to any of us, but children under 14 and the elderly are most vulnerable. The risk of falling, in particular, rises sharply with age, according to the American Academy of Family Physicians. More than half of all falls that happen at home are due to hazards such as poorly lit stairways, notes Judy Stevens, PhD, an epidemiologist for the CDC Injury Center in Atlanta. But most of these obstacles are quite easy to fix, once you know where to find them. Here's what to look for.

1 DON'T SLIP UP!

You trip, you skid, you lose your footing—you look down as though the floor is to blame. One way to avoid these awkward accidental ballets is to wear shoes and slippers with rubber soles at all times. Also, use throw rugs with non-skid backing, or put tape on the bottom to hold them in place. And don't wait to clean up spills—wipe them up as soon as they happen.

2 THINK BEFORE YOU STORE

Place items within arm's reach rather than up so high that you're teetering on your toes to retrieve them. If you need a boost, use a step ladder or ladder. Chairs aren't made to be stood upon!

3 REMOVE STUMBLING BLOCKS

Common pathways should be clear of clutter. Pick up laundry, books, shoes, toys, and other items that tend to

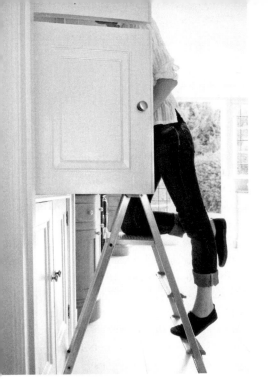

bed rails, safety gates, outlet covers, and other safeguards. Move chairs and other furniture that provides easy access to windows. And keep anything small out of reach. If it can fit through a small parts tester (about the size of a cardboard toilet paper tube), than it's considered a choking hazard.

6 READ PRODUCT LABELS

If you see words like "Caution," "Warning," "Danger" or "Keep out of reach of children," take them seriously. Store these items—which include medications, cosmetics, and cleaning products—where children can't get to them, ideally behind child safety locks, Appy says.

7 GET A GRASP ON THINGS

Railings should run the full length of both sides of a staircase. If you have a child or an elderly person in your home who's at special risk for falling, install grab rails in the shower as well as bedrails.

8 BE PREPARED

Post a list of emergency phone numbers by every phone. The list should include numbers for your doctor, police department, and the poison control hotline (800-222-1222). And have a first-aid kit on hand. Check the contents once a year and replace items that have expired.

congregate on floors and stairs. Other possible booby traps are hanging wires and cords. If you can't move them, have an electrician install outlets in safer places.

4 LIGHTEN THINGS UP

Your home should be well lit so that family members and guests can navigate hallways and stairways without incident. Night lights will make nocturnal visits to the bathroom and kitchen much safer. It's also a good idea to keep a flashlight near your bed in case of a power outage.

5 GET A TODDLER'S-EYE VIEW

Having a toddler in your home requires extra precautions. "Even before a child starts to crawl or attempts those first steps, you need to get down on your hands and knees and take a second look at the safety of your home from the toddler's point-of-view," says Meri-K Appy, president of the Home Safety Council. "Inspect each room to spot the hazards that need to be fixed, and then fix them." Install window guards,

your list

6 steps to fire-proof your home

mini LIST

Extinguish with care

Portable extinguishers are an extremely valuable first line of defense for most (though not all) home fires. You may use an extinguisher when:

1. You've alerted other occupants and called the fire department.

2. The fire is small and contained, like in a cooking pot or trash can.

3. You're safe from toxic smoke.

4. The fire isn't blocking your escape route and your instincts tell you that you're safe.

Note that all four of these criteria must be met. If they aren't, the US Fire Administration advises against using an extinguisher. Instead, evacuate your home immediately and use a cell phone to call for help.

YOU LOVE TO light candles in your living room because of the aroma and atmosphere they create. But let's suppose one of them gets knocked over and catches a magazine. How long do you think you'd have to get to safety? According to a survey of over 1,000 people, over 88% said that they'd have less than 30 minutes to escape, with 25% indicating they'd have at least 10 minutes. In reality, a living room fire can turn deadly in just 2 minutes—sometimes less.

This isn't meant to put you off of burning candles (though, honestly, dampening the flame may not be a bad idea, especially if you have kids or pets in your home). Our purpose is to illustrate how easily something seemingly innocuous can turn disastrous in an instant—and how a few simple precautions can go a long way in protecting you and your loved ones. Here's how you can keep those home fires burning—safely.

1 PUT SAFETY ON THE MENU

Cooking fires account for 40% of all home fires. You can reduce the risk simply by being there, says Lorraine Carli, vice president of communications for the National Fire Protection Agency. If you are frying, broiling, or grilling food and you need to walk away, turn off the stove first. If you are baking, roasting, boiling, or simmering, check your food regularly and don't leave while you're cooking. Move anything that could catch fire away from the oven. Potholders, mitts, towels, curtains, and food cartons all present a fire risk around the stovetop, Carli says. Also, dress for the task at hand. Wear tight-fitting or rolled-up sleeves while working around the stove. "Only about 1% of cooking fires are caused by clothing catching on fire, but these clothing fires account for about 12% of deaths," Carli notes.

2 LAUNDER WITH CARE

One of every 23 residential fires starts in a washing machine or dryer, with dryers accounting for 92%. Many of these fires could be prevented if the appliances were kept clean. Remove lint after each load of laundry and regularly check the outdoor vent to make sure that it's free from obstruction. Never run the dryer while you aren't home or you're sleeping. If clothing comes into contact with a flammable liquid such as alcohol, paint thinner, or cooking oil, lay it aside to dry before laundering. Finally, have your dryer serviced by professionals as needed, especially if you have a gas model, Carli advises.

3 PUT SPACE HEATERS IN THEIR PLACE

If you use any type of fuel-burning appliance to heat your home, be especially careful to avoid two of the most common winter dangers: fire and carbon monoxide poisoning, says Meri-K Appy, president of the Home Safety Council. (For information on CO, see page 162.)

Keep space heaters at least 3 feet away from furniture, curtains, beds, and anything else that can burn. Turn them off before falling asleep or leaving the room. And check to confirm that your heater has undergone testing by an independent lab, as indicated by an ETL, UL, or CSA seal (usually located on the bottom of the appliance).

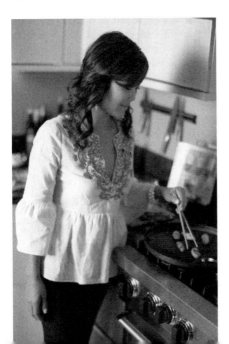

4 FOLLOW SAFE CINDER RULES

Many chimney and fireplace fires are triggered by a buildup of creosote, an oily combustible byproduct of the incomplete burning of wood. The easiest way to prevent this buildup is to burn wood completely. Only use seasoned hardwoods, such as oak or ash, in your fireplace. The wood should be split, stacked, and allowed to dry for 12 months. Use sturdy screens and doors to keep embers from escaping. And have your fireplace inspected by a professional chimney sweep once a year.

5 BE ON ALERT

A working smoke alarm cuts your chances of losing your life to a fire by half. Install alarms in every bedroom, outside of sleeping areas, and on every level of your home. Test them at least once a month and replace batteries at least once a year, the National Fire Protection Association recommends.

6 CHECK THE EXTINGUISHER

Install your fire extinguisher in a place where you can get to it quickly and easily. Keep the pressure at the recommended level. If you see any signs of damage, like dents or rust, replace the device, the US Fire Administration suggests.

your list

7 steps to organize your home

mini LIST

Tools for tidiness

The following items don't cost much, but they're invaluable for helping to keep your house in order:

- **Plastic bins.** Use them to store off-season clothing. They can be stashed under the bed or in the closet.

- **Hooks.** Encourage family members to use them for coats, sweaters, hats, purses, book bags, and other accoutrements that tend to amass on the backs of chairs or the floor.

- **Label maker.** Making clear to everyone what belongs where will help maintain organization.

- **Dishpans.** Use them for kid's stuff such as coloring books and crayons, miniature cars and trucks, and dolls and clothing. Place them on shelves for easy access, or stow them under a child's bed.

THE WORD "CLUTTER" means different things to different people. For some, it's when their DVDs aren't in alphabetical order. For others, it's when they can no longer see their carpet. But when does clutter reach crisis proportions? "If you can't straighten up your house in 20 minutes when a guest calls to say that she's coming over, than you have a problem," says professional organizer Barbara Hemphill, coauthor of *Love It or Lose It: Living Clutter-Free Forever*.

If you feel paralyzed by the amount of clutter around your home, your best strategy is to attack it piecemeal. Commit to spending at least 20 to 30 minutes on uncluttering each day, but no more than an hour," says organizing pro Donna Smallin, author of *The One Minute Organizer Plain and Simple*. "After an hour, you won't be so fresh, and your decision-making ability may falter." Focus on one room, or one part of a room, at a time, so you can see your progress. And once you've untangled the clutter, you can address the disorderly conduct that started the whole mess.

1 SPILL IT

Gather up those mysterious boxes in the attic, the junk drawers, and the odds-and-ends bags. Your mission is to divide their contents into three piles: Keep (items you use regularly), Store (items you want to keep but don't need to have handy), and Remove (items you can toss or donate). As you assess each item, ask yourself whether it is useful or beautiful or it has some value. If you can't answer yes to at least one of these questions, then the item belongs on the Remove pile. If you just can't make up your mind about something, set it aside for now. Then if you don't miss it after 60 days, find another home for it. Also hang on to any baskets, bowls, and other containers that could be used for storage.

2 MAKE ROOM FOR THE KEEPERS

Store these items in cabinets and drawers close to where you'll use or need them. For example, put pens in the home office, guest towels in the linen closet, bread baskets in the kitchen cabinet. Items that are called upon daily, like the coffee maker and cotton balls, merit counter space. Those that are pulled out only occasionally can be moved to harder-to-reach cabinets and drawers.

3 FIND NEW PURPOSE

If you came across baskets and other containers during your initial search-and-rescue mission, now is the time to put them to use. Set a few in each room to house small related items. In the living room, for example, perhaps one basket can hold pens, crossword puzzles, and reading glasses, while another is reserved for the remote and the TV viewing guide.

4 SAY GOODBYE TO THE REMOVE PILE

Before setting curbside, though, consider whether the items in this pile may find new life with someone else. For example, organizations such as Goodwill and the Salvation Army are always looking for furniture, clothing, toys, and books. "I donate to a domestic violence center," Hemphill says. "What they don't use they ship overseas." Anything that is broken, outdated, or missing parts or that has little value can be trashed or recycled, Smallin says.

5 TAME THE PAPER

Coupon flyers, old newspapers, and magazines can quickly clutter your living space. Get in the habit of tossing or shredding paper that you don't need or want. Remove your name from mailing lists and cancel subscriptions for magazines that you can read at the library for free. Elect to receive bills as email reminders rather than through the postal service, Smallin suggests. For any documents that you want to hang on to, consider scanning them and storing them electronically.

6 KEEP IT UP

Controlling clutter is an ongoing process, according to the experts at the National Association of Professional Organizers. "Think about it as 'being organized' or 'staying organized,' instead of 'getting organized,'" they suggest.

7 INVOLVE EVERYONE

You can lead by example, but maintaining order must be a group effort. Meet weekly with family members to discuss de-cluttering assignments. Staying organized runs in the family.

your list

7 documents to keep safe

Online personal health records could save your life in an emergency, says David Katz, MD, MPH, director of the Prevention Research Center at Yale University School of Medicine. Most sites encrypt data for security. Here are a few to choose from:

- **Mayo Clinic Health Manager,** healthmanager. mayoclinic.com. This free site also offers information on the latest treatments for various conditions.

- **Google Health,** google.com/health. Store health records and share them with others for free, and print out a wallet-size profile to keep with you in case of an emergency.

- **Passport MD,** passportmd.com. Members receive medication reminders sent to their phones.

CERTAIN DOCUMENTS INSPIRE the pack rat in all of us: gift receipts, instruction manuals (even for gadgets we no longer have), and—the granddaddy of all paper piles—income taxes. If you can't easily put your fingers on the one document that you really need because of the dense file or mountain of paper that it's buried in, then you're probably hanging on to more than you should.

It might help to think of your home as a small business. Records should be retained for tax purposes as well as for proof of payment and ownership. Other documents are preserved for crises like death, fire, or theft. These papers carry enormous personal and financial weight, so purging them once they've outlived their usefulness can be an uneasy task. But take comfort: If you lose or shred something by mistake, the document probably can be recreated, although typically at some expense.

To make the paper trail less rocky, follow these guidelines when deciding what to keep and for how long.

1 PERSONAL RECORDS

Birth certificates, burial lot deeds, and wills should travel with you wherever you go. Other documents that should tag along:

- Baptismal record: Use this as evidence of birthdate if you don't have a birth certificate on hand.
- Diplomas and education records: You'll need these as proof of education and attendance.
- Divorce decree: This will clear legal requirements in the event of remarriage.
- Medical record: Keep a medical history—including immunization, major illness, and surgery—for every family member and update it as necessary.

Store all of these vital papers in a safe deposit box at your bank or in a fire-proof safe in your home. It's a good idea to keep a separate list of all of these documents and their location, just in case someone else needs to access them on your behalf.

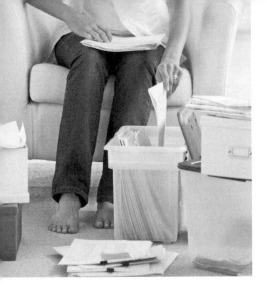

5 HOUSEHOLD AND CREDIT CARD BILLS

Once they're paid, there's no reason to hold on to these unless they show tax-deductible expenses. Some people prefer to keep certain bills until they can check that they've received credit for payment on the next month's statement.

6 PAY STUBS

File away your pay stubs until you receive your W-2 form at the end of the year. Once you confirm that the amounts match, you can discard the stubs.

7 LIEN DOCUMENTS

Keep real estate deeds, titles, mortgage, and other lien documents for the duration of ownership. If you sell property, the IRS suggests retaining the settlement records for 7 years for tax purposes.

your list

_____

_____

_____

_____

_____

_____

_____

_____

_____

_____

_____

_____

_____

_____

_____

2 TAX RETURNS

The Internal Revenue Service suggests that once you've filed your income tax return, you should hang on to all of the documents for as long as you can file an amended return or as long as the IRS can assess additional taxes. Keep in mind that your taxes can be audited for up to 3 years after they've been filed. If the IRS suspects that you've underreported your taxes by 25% or more, they can assess additional taxes as long as it's within 6 years of the original filing date.

3 BANK STATEMENTS

Some experts suggest shredding bank statements after a few months, while others advise storing them for 7 years for tax purposes. Find out how long your bank retains financial records. If you can order a statement when you need it, you may decide to purge your copies after a couple of months.

4 CANCELED CHECKS AND DEPOSIT SLIPS

Keep these, as well as ATM slips and credit card receipts, until you verify them on your monthly account statement. Once you confirm that they've been recorded accurately, shred them unless you need them for tax purposes or as proof of payment for items under warranty.

8 best and worst places to store your stuff

my favorite...
Sniff Test

Maureen Donovan, PhD, professor, College of Pharmacy, University of Iowa

According to Donovan, one of the easiest and quickest ways to tell if medication is past its prime is to give it a sniff test. "Some drugs smell differently when they go bad. They may produce an odor that's hard to ignore," she says. "For example, aspirin reacts to moisture in the air by creating acetic acid, which smells like vinegar."

IF YOU'VE WALKED through grass or dirt, check your shoes by the door, please! They may be made for walking, but not to your bedroom closet. The soles are steeped in contaminants and allergens seeking a place to squat.

Usually we don't give much thought to where we stow things—but perhaps we should. Choosing the wrong storage spot may shorten the shelf life of some items and increase the health risks of others. Consider these words of wisdom when deciding where your belongings belong, and where they don't.

1 TOOTHBRUSHES

The worst place: The bathroom sink. It's too close to the toilet. According to germ expert Chuck Gerba, PhD, professor of environmental microbiology at the University of Arizona, every square inch of a typical toilet bowl is home to 3.2 million microbes. With every flush, toilet funk can be propelled as far as 6 feet, showering the sink with bacteria.

The best place: Behind closed doors. "Unless you like rinsing your mouth with toilet water, keep your toothbrush in a medicine cabinet or a nearby cupboard," Gerba suggests.

2 MEDICINE

The worst place: The medicine cabinet. A steamy bathroom can reach up to 100°F, which could affect the potency of many common medications. For instance, the effectiveness of Lipitor—a common cholesterol drug—could be compromised at a temperature of 77°F or higher.

The best place: A cool, dry place like a pantry or hall closet.

3 COFFEE

The worst place: The refrigerator or freezer. Many people think that cold storage helps to preserve the freshness and flavor of coffee. Every time you retrieve it, however, the resulting temperature fluctuation produces condensation. "The moisture leeches out flavor. It's like brewing a cup of coffee each time," explains John McGregor, PhD, professor in the department of food science and human nutrition at Clemson University.

The best place: In an opaque, airtight container that's stored either on the kitchen counter or in the pantry.

4 SHOES

The worst place: The bedroom closet. Traipsing through your home with shoes that you've been wearing outside is a great way to track in pollen and other allergens, as well as contaminants like lawn chemicals.

The best place: By the door. Store them in baskets or another container by the entryway. If your shoes stay off the lawn, they can make their way to the bedroom—but only if they're carried.

5 HANDBAGS

The worst place: Any surface normally used for food preparation or eating. Handbags carry more than wallets; they're terrific microbe magnets. When Gerba and his team of researchers swabbed the bottoms of purses, they found 10,000 bacteria per inch. Even worse, one-third of the bags tested positive for fecal bacteria! It's not surprising, though, when you think about all of those nasty spots where we park our handbags: bus seats, restaurant floors, bathroom stalls.

The best place: A drawer, a chair—anyplace except where food is prepared or eaten, Gerba advises.

6 BATTERIES

The worst place: The refrigerator. According to Duracell, cold temperatures affect the integrity of household batteries. Hot temperatures impact performance as well.

The best place: In a dry environment at room temperature. Make sure, too, that the contact surfaces aren't touching.

7 TELEVISION

The worst place: Wherever you dine. Research shows that TV watching encourages mindless eating. In one Canadian study, for example, eating dinner while parked in front of a television had a negative effect on fruit and vegetable consumption as well as overall nutrition.

The best place: Up or down a flight of stairs from your kitchen. When snacks take more effort to get to, you'll be less likely to munch while watching.

8 NIGHTTIME READING LIGHT

The worst place: Overhead. These fixtures emit a relatively bright light—enough to significantly delay the body's secretion of the hormone melatonin, according to research. That can set you up for a restless night since melatonin levels are a major cue for your body to prepare for sleep.

The best place: Anywhere but the bedroom. A better lighting alternative is a lower-powered light clipped to your novel. It provides enough light to read but leaves the room dark enough for your brain to transition into sleep mode.

your list

_____

_____

_____

_____

_____

_____

_____

_____

_____

_____

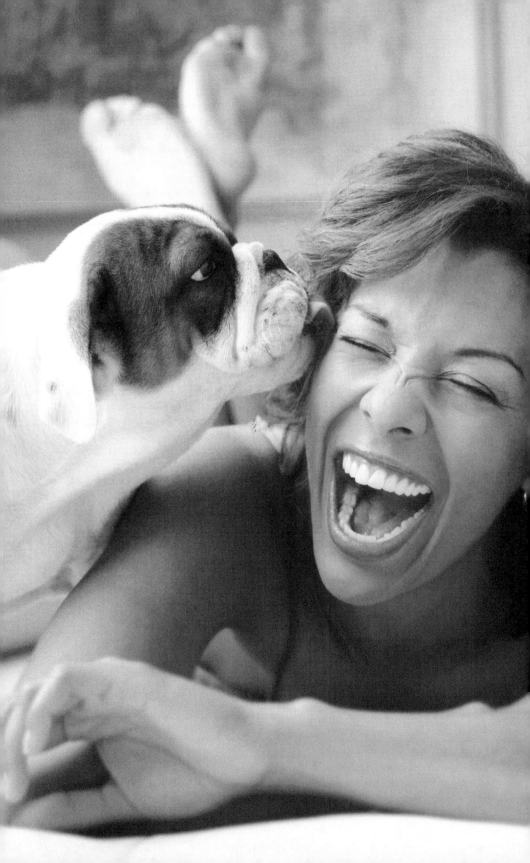

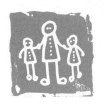

chapter 7 life

10 big ideas for the 21st century

facts & figures

29.2
years

Increase in life
expectancy between
1900 and 1999,
according to the
Centers for Disease
Control and
Prevention.

IT'S UNDENIABLE THAT the 20th century produced some amazing medical breakthroughs. From medicines and vaccines to diagnostic techniques and surgical procedures, these pioneering advances have dramatically improved our chances of surviving a major medical crisis.

So what can we expect for the next 100 years? To find out, we polled some of America's foremost medical minds for their opinions on what they perceive as the next big ideas to emerge from medical science. Here's what they said.

1 HEALTH ON THE GO

Today's doctors routinely order blood glucose, blood pressure, and cholesterol screenings for their patients. Imagine being able to check those numbers yourself, then upload and send them to your doctor for him or her to assess. A company called Ideal Life (IdealLifeOnline.com) is already making a series of wireless-enabled instruments to do exactly that.

2 LABORATORY-GROWN ORGANS

"We are on the precipice of being able to construct complex organs, fabricated from organic matrices to which a patient's cells can be added," says Thom Lobe, MD, founder and medical director of the Beneveda Medical Group in Beverly Hills. So new bladders, hearts, intestines, and other structures can be generated to replace those that have been damaged by trauma or disease.

3 A BETTER BRAIN

Currently brain trauma is devastating and irreversible. But will this always be the case? "In the future, we will see the development of sophisticated computer chips that are part neural tissue and part semiconductor," Lobe predicts. "They'll perform certain brain functions that have been disrupted by trauma, tumor, or stroke."

4 A CURE FOR ALZHEIMER'S

There's already significant evidence that Alzheimer's disease is hereditary or caused by cell transformation, according to Thomas Royer, MD, president and CEO of

Christus Health in Irving, Texas. "Knowledge from genotyping should permit us to successfully develop a process to inhibit the gene transformation," he says.

5 BABIES ON DEMAND

Women who postpone starting families until later in life soon may have more options. With the proliferation of egg freezing technology, it's possible for women to safely have healthy babies even after they're past their peak in fertility, says John Jain, MD, a former researcher at the University of Southern California and founder of Santa Monica Fertility Specialists.

6 WIDESPREAD USE OF ALTERNATIVE THERAPIES

If you're already using these therapies in your self-care, you're ahead of the curve—but the curve is catching up. "Complementary and alternative medicine that has been traditionally scoffed at will be better understood and more widely accepted by insurers, traditionally trained physicians, and consumers," Lobe says. "These types of therapy will be integrated into current practice."

7 A DIABETES RESOLUTION

Doctors may come to rely on gastric bypass surgery as a treatment not only for obesity but also for type 2 diabetes. According to a review of 621 studies conducted between 1990 and 2006, 86.6% of patients who underwent gastric bypass saw their diabetes improve or resolve completely. The review appeared in the March 2009 issue of the *American Journal of Medicine*.

8 DIGITAL HOUSE CALLS

You can get a full checkup from your doctor without leaving your home. "Connected Care combines state-of-the-art video technology and health resources to greatly expand physicians' reach into rural, urban, and underserved areas," notes Reed Tuckson, MD, executive vice president and chief of medical affairs for UnitedHealth Group. "It is linking patients to physicians and specialists who could be hundreds of miles away."

9 SURGICAL ROBOTS

This technology isn't new, but its use will expand in the years ahead. "From my and other people's research, I'm convinced that robots will enable abdominal surgery through almost any natural orifice, such as the mouth, vagina, rectum, or even bladder," says Monika Hagen, MD, a researching surgeon in the field of new technologies for minimally invasive surgery in San Diego. "This revolution will lead to surgery that is much less invasive and that doesn't leave visible scars."

10 AN END TO AGING?

Studies at the cellular and even chromosomal level are yielding a new understanding of how we age. Future discoveries may allow us to slow or even stop the aging process. "The telomere on your chromosomes controls how fast your cells divide and thus age," says Michael Hall, MD, creator of the Longevity Anti-Aging Center in Miami Beach. "They can be given new life and kept healthy with the enzyme telomerase."

your list

_____

_____

_____

_____

_____

8 doable New Year's resolutions

mini LIST

7 ways to eat well

Ann G. Kulze, MD, founder and CEO of Just Wellness, LLC, and author of *Dr. Ann's 10-Step Diet*, recommends the following nutrition resolutions.

- Replace other oils with olive oil.

- Give up refined grain products like white bread and white rice in favor of 100% whole grains.

- Reduce your consumption of empty liquid calories such as sodas, fruit drinks, and sports drinks.

- Eat more beans; few foods are as nutritious and easy to prepare.

- Never skip a meal— especially breakfast.

- Choose only real, whole foods.

- Eat a small handful of nuts every day (any type will do, though almonds and walnuts offer the most healthful benefits).

IN THEORY, NEW Year's resolutions are a fabulous idea. After all, what better way to start the New Year than with a fresh outlook on life?

In practice, this annual ritual has become a bit of a joke, to the point that people make bets about how long their friends' and loved ones' resolutions are going to last. For some, it's gotten so futile that they've stopped making resolutions altogether.

The problem, says David L. Katz, MD, MPH, director of the Yale Griffin Prevention Research Center in Derby, Connecticut, and author of *The Way to Eat*, is that many resolutions are unrealistic and poorly executed. "Most resolutions involve inspiration but no preparation," he says. "For long-term success, a detailed and sustainable action plan is key."

With help from our experts, we've put together a list of resolutions for you to try. Many are a spin on the usual resolutions, but with tips for making them stick. You needn't wait for the New Year to give these a test drive!

1 CHANGE YOUR OUTLOOK ON HEALTH

Instead of seeing it as all-or-nothing, Rallie McAllister, MD, MPH, a family physician in Lexington, Kentucky, and founder and medical director of *The Mommy MD Guides*, suggests viewing health as a continuum. "Every decision that I make moves me closer to one end of the continuum (good health) or the other (poor health)," she says. "For instance, drinking a soda would move me in the wrong direction, while drinking a glass of water would move me in the right direction. By making small, positive decisions, I move closer and closer to good health."

2 INTEGRATE EXERCISE

For most people, exercise is an add-on, something that they do if they can find time. It's much easier to accommodate if you find ways to incorporate activity into your daily routine. "Climbing the stairs to the third floor takes just a minute longer than waiting for the elevator.

Likewise, jogging to the mailbox at the end of my driveway takes a minute or two, but it's so much better for me than simply leaning out my car window as I drive by," McAllister says. "When we find reasons to stay active throughout the day, we can afford to miss an exercise session every now and then."

3 SAY GOODBYE TO FAD DIETS

Losing weight is a favorite resolution . . . which may help explain why so many diets fail. It's fine to have weight loss as a goal, but instead of following the latest diet craze, focus your efforts on eating healthfully, says Nadia Rodman, RD, registered dietitian for Curves Health Clubs and Fitness Centers for Women. For a few nutrition pointers, see the Mini-List.

4 HEAD BACK TO THE KITCHEN

"Have you noticed that kitchens are getting fancier and fancier, yet fewer and fewer people are actually using them?" Rodman says. The beauty of resolving to do more of your own cooking is that you gain more control over the nutritional quality of your meals. "Prepare your own food from fresh ingredients," Rodman suggests. "You will save calories and money, and you will be healthier for it."

5 UNPLUG DAILY

Thanks to modern electronics, we're switched on and tuned in 24/7—it's ratcheting up our stress level as a result. "Spend an hour, 10 hours, or a full day without your cell phone, Blackberry, computer, or games," urges Ashley Koff, RD, a registered dietitian in Los Angeles. "What will happen if someone can't reach you or you can't reach someone else at a moment's notice? Where will your imagination take you?"

6 CONQUER CLUTTER

Another way to reduce your stress level is to work on clearing out the clutter in your home. "Living in the midst of clutter saps your energy," says Thom Lobe, MD. "Clean up your mess, and it will open up your life for more positive energy." For tips on sifting through your stuff and creating a more organized home, see page 170.

7 GET YOUR FINANCIAL HOUSE IN ORDER

There is no time like the present to lay out a plan for saving more and spending less. To get started, Jim Roberts, PhD, professor of marketing at Baylor University in Waco, Texas, recommends establishing an emergency fund of $2,500 and reducing your credit card use for an entire year.

8 EMBRACE GENEROSITY

Few things are as easy or provide as much instant gratification as donating time or money to people in need. "Give away 1% more of your income than you did last year; volunteer at a food bank in the middle of summer; go out of your way for someone who seemingly has nothing to offer you," says Kathy LeMay, founder, president, and CEO of Raising Change, a fundraising organization. "When you unleash your generosity potential, your life will be the better for it. Slowly, we'll begin to create the world that we know is possible."

your list ————
————
————
————
————
————
————

9 ways to make the most of your day

my favorite...
Time to Exercise

Rallie McAllister, MD, MPH, a family physician

The best time to exercise is a topic of much debate among experts, but McAllister makes a case for working out first thing in the morning. "Try to exercise on an empty stomach—before breakfast if you can," she says. "That way, you're more likely to pull calories from fat stores and lose body fat more quickly."

One time not to exercise is right before going to bed. Physical activity stimulates the release of endorphins, which may keep you awake.

IN LIFE, TIMING can be everything—and that holds true even for your daily routine. When you do certain things at certain times of day, you can be more efficient and effective—and you can feel better for it.

The secret is to know your body well enough that you can set your daily calendar to your own internal clock. "Try to schedule your activities so that your body rhythms fully support you," advises Rallie McAllister, MD, MPH, a family physician. "For instance, if you feel energized, motivated, and mentally sharp first thing in the morning, tackle your most challenging tasks—such as writing a report or creating a business plan—during this time." On the other hand, if you tend to feel sluggish after lunch, steer clear of any activity that demands a lot of brain power. Instead, you might want to do something that gets you up and moving, McAllister says.

While your body should be your ultimate guide, our experts do have a few suggestions as far as the best times of the day for handling certain tasks. Here's what they had to say.

1 THE BEST TIME TO ... WEIGH YOURSELF

First thing in the morning, after you go to the bathroom but before you take a shower or eat breakfast, advises Erin Palinski, RD, a registered dietitian in New York City. And you should be naked when you step on the scale. "This will give you your most accurate body weight on a day-to-day basis," she says.

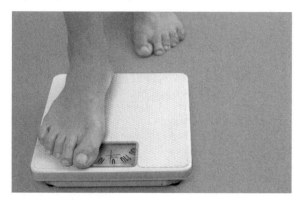

2 THE BEST TIME TO . . . EAT BREAKFAST

Every day, and within an hour of waking. "Eating breakfast can jump-start your metabolism, helping you to stay at a healthy body weight," Palinski says. "It also has been shown to help regulate appetite and prevent overeating later in the day."

3 THE BEST TIME TO . . . EAT OTHER MEALS

Throughout the day—but they should be smaller than the standard three squares. "Small meals keep your metabolism going and therefore help you reach your fitness goals faster," notes James Rouse, ND, a naturopathic physician in Denver. Choosing the right foods is essential. For example, a healthy midday snack would be a handful of almonds, string cheese, and yogurt rather than a bag of potato chips and a bottle of cola.

4 THE BEST TIME TO . . . EAT YOUR LAST MEAL OF THE DAY

At least 2½ hours before bed, and preferably 3½. "Eating right before you lie down increases your chances of experiencing heartburn and GERD (gastroesophageal reflux disease)," McAllister says.

5 THE BEST TIME TO . . . TAKE A MULTIVITAMIN

At lunch. While most people take their multivitamins first thing in the morning, Ashley Koff, RD, says that you may get more benefit by taking it at lunchtime instead for a boost of afternoon energy.

6 THE BEST TIME TO . . . GO GROCERY SHOPPING

Try 9 o'clock in the evening, if not later. When you're out this late, you're likely to have the store mostly to yourself, says Dana Korey, a professional organizer and founder of Away with Clutter, a professional organizing service in Southern California.

7 THE BEST TIME TO . . . TACKLE BIG TASKS

First thing in the morning. "Your mind is clear; your body is free from any strain and stress; and you generally have a good outlook," Rouse says. "Try to make big decisions when your body and mind are in the right place."

8 THE BEST TIME TO . . . GIVE A PRESENTATION

Any time except right after lunch. If your audience is coming back after a big meal, they may fall asleep on you, Korey says.

9 THE BEST TIME TO . . . GET SOME SLEEP

When the sun goes down. "Darkness improves the depth of sleep and thus allows your body the best recovery," Koff says.

your list

7 ways to make the most of your week

my favorite...
Day of the Week to Fly

Richard B. Chess, managing partner of Chess Law Firm, Richmond, Virginia (and a frequent flier)

Chess recommends flying Sunday night, Tuesday morning, or Thursday night. "These are some of the least busy times at an airport, so the usual lines, crowds, and congestion are gone, making the skies truly friendly," he says. The flights tend to be emptier, so aisle seats are available, and bags seem less likely to get lost. Plus, planning your flight for one of these times keeps you from becoming trapped in what Chess describes as "hell on earth—the Atlanta airport on a late Friday afternoon during a thundershower!"

SOME DAYS SEEM to go perfectly, while others leave us thinking that we should have stayed in bed. Part of the reason is timing: Just as certain times of day are better suited to certain tasks, so are certain days of the week. It's true whether we're running errands or planning something bigger, like finding a new job.

As you set your schedule for the week ahead, peruse the following list to see whether you might better correlate the task at hand with the appropriate day. Who knows? It could make all of the difference in the outcome.

1 BEST DAY TO . . . ASK FOR A RAISE: MONDAY

It may seem counterintuitive, but according to Peter Handal, CEO of Dale Carnegie Training, a corporate, leadership and sales training school, you have your best chance of getting your supervisor's undivided attention on Monday. "Bosses and managers typically feel more rested and fresh from the weekend, so they are more likely to take time to listen to your case and not be preoccupied with other employee and client obligations," Handal says. You should plan ahead, though, by scheduling the meeting at least a week in advance. And try for a time slot early in the morning rather than late in the day.

2 BEST DAY TO . . . SEE THE DOCTOR: WEDNESDAY

Doctor's offices are slammed on Monday, and sometimes the rush can spill into Tuesday, as well. By Wednesday, things have settled down, and you can get the doctor's undivided attention. "If you can get an appointment first thing in the morning, the unexpected time delays have not had time to add up, and you will likely be in and out quickly," says D.J. Verret, MD, an assistant clinical professor at the University of Texas Southwestern Medical School in Dallas.

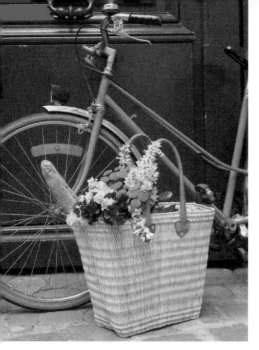

make sure that the calories taken in at your favorite restaurant are accounted for in advance by calories out."

6 BEST DAY TO . . . GROCERY SHOP: SUNDAY AND WEDNESDAY

Ashley Koff, RD, recommends shopping twice weekly—once on Sunday and again on Wednesday. That way you're certain to get the freshest of the fresh ingredients, including fruits, vegetables, and herbs and spices. Supermarkets do tend to be crowded on weekends, so you may want to plan your shopping for later in the evening—or simply steel yourself for long lines.

7 BEST DAY TO . . . EXERCISE: SUNDAY AND MONDAY

You should be squeezing in at least 30 minutes of physical activity most days of the week. But Koff says that by making a point to work out on Sunday and Monday, you increase your chances of following suit the rest of the week.

3 BEST DAY TO . . . TAKE OFF: MONDAY OR FRIDAY

Why? You get a long weekend, of course! But there are other good reasons, too. "Taking a vacation day in the middle of the week is hard not only for you but for your colleagues who must pick up the slack," Handal says. "By taking Monday or Friday, you can sort your workload throughout the rest of the week."

4 BEST DAY TO . . . LOOK FOR A NEW JOB: SATURDAY

If you're still employed, of course, you don't want to be caught exploring new prospects on your current employer's time. Plus, "the nation's newspapers upload their new job listings on Friday nights," says Robin Ryan, a career counselor and author of *Over 40 and You're Hired!*

5 BEST DAY TO . . . GO OUT TO DINNER: SATURDAY

Why? The restaurant may be busier on Saturday, but David L. Katz, MD, MPH, says it's still his top pick. "It can be a treat to relish, rather than a routine that under-mines your health," he says. "Plus, you have time on Saturday to get exercise to

your list ———
—————————————————
—————————————————
—————————————————
—————————————————
—————————————————
—————————————————
—————————————————
—————————————————
—————————————————
—————————————————

8 must-haves for any emergency

my favorite...
Website

Becky Marquis, acting director of FEMA's Ready Campaign

The Federal Emergency Management Agency (FEMA) wants your family to be prepared in the event of an emergency, which is why they've launched the Ready Campaign. "On our website, you'll find all of the facts that you need to handle an emergency situation," Marquis says. "We provide tips and information on how to prepare, particularly the top things to have at home for emergencies." For more information, visit www.ready.gov.

ALL OF US can learn a lesson from the Boy Scout credo "Be prepared." How well you weather any emergency, big or small, depends in large part on how well you plan for it.

"In the event of a truly major event, public emergency response organizations will be overwhelmed and unable to respond to every situation and need," notes Chris Cowles, marketing manager for Safer Systems, a company that specializes in chemical emergency response solutions. "Therefore, individuals and families must be prepared to take care of themselves and their neighbors until outside help can arrive—which could be days in certain circumstances. People need to become their own 'first responders.'"

By the very nature of an emergency, you can't predict exactly what will happen or when. To be prepared, then, you'll want a stash of supplies that are versatile enough to be useful in a variety of situations. You may need to invest in some items—but your and your family's welfare is worth the expense.

1 FOOD, WATER, AND MEDICINE
You never know how long you'll need to stay in your home, which is why having plenty of canned and packaged foods and bottles of water is important, says Kelly Rouba, senior manager for EAD & Associates, an emergency management and special needs consulting firm in New York City. Keep a manual can opener handy, in case you are without power. Get extras of any essential medications, too, says Renee Grasso of Be Safe Plus, LLC in Lake Hiawatha, New Jersey.

2 FLASHLIGHT AND RADIO
These gadgets are no-brainers. In addition to the battery-operated kind, though, look for models that can be hand cranked. "They're great backups for when the batteries in traditional flashlights or radios fail," Grasso says.

3 CASH AND ESSENTIAL DOCUMENTS

We live in a credit card world, but we can't be certain that plastic will work in an emergency. That's why Rouba recommends having cash on hand. "Just keep as much as you are comfortable with, in small denominations," she says.

Along with your cash, store any essential documents that you don't carry with you every day, such as passports and Social Security cards.

4 IMPORTANT PHONE NUMBERS

Like credit cards, a cell phone may or may not work in an emergency. So don't count on being able to access important phone numbers at the press of a button. Instead, make a separate phone list. "It should include your doctors, your pharmacist, any care or service providers and medical supply companies, and your network of emergency contacts, which should include a friend or relative in your region as well as someone who's long distance," Rouba says.

5 A FAMILY CONTACT PLAN

Considering the dynamic of the modern American family, chances are good that your clan won't be in the same place when disaster strikes. "You need to have a plan for yourself and your family, so everyone knows whom to contact in the event of an emergency," Cowles says.

6 FIRE SAFETY EQUIPMENT

Most homes have smoke detectors, but they should also be equipped with fire extinguishers on every level of the home, as well as fire safety ladders on the upper levels. "These ladders provide an alternative escape route when traditional routes are blocked by smoke, fire, or debris," Grasso says. "They are essential for all two-story homes and above."

7 FIRST-AID KIT

With a well-stocked first-aid kit, you'll be able to render immediate care for illnesses and injuries until emergency personnel can reach you. The American Red Cross has posted a list of essential first-aid supplies on its website: www.redcross.org.

8 A "GO" BAG

Some emergencies may leave you home-bound, while others require a quick escape. When that's the case, you'll want a bag that's packed with essentials and ready to go on a moment's notice. Grasso suggests that your bag contain many of the items discussed here, as well as a change of clothes for each family member and blankets.

your list

9 tools every homeowner needs

facts & figures

$200

Cost to clean and declutter a home.

$1,700

Perceived increase in home value, according to HomeGain.com, a blog for the real estate community.

NOT ALL OF us are as handy as Bob Vila, but even the most novice DIY-er can handle a surprising amount of home repairs with some research, elbow grease—and the right tools.

As you'll see, you needn't drop a lot of cash to assemble your home tool kit. Most of the tools cost just a few dollars at your local hardware store or home center. Nor do you require advanced carpentry skills to use them; with these tools, a little bit of common sense goes a long way.

You can tackle most basic repairs with the tool collection presented here.

1 ALL-IN-ONE PAINTER'S TOOL

This hand tool—which looks a little like a putty knife with a pointed end—is indispensable for a variety of home projects, not just painting. "You can use it to scrape off old paint and caulk, fill holes with spackle, open paint cans, clean paint rollers, pry off old trim, remove old floor tiles (in tandem with a hammer), and knock in nails," says Dean Bennett, president of Dean Bennett Design and Construction in Castle Rock, Colorado. "Many models have an attachment for a screwdriver. For around $5 to $12, it's a remarkably versatile tool."

2 SAW AND SCREWDRIVER COMBINATION TOOL

With this hybrid, you get a selection of screwdriver bits as well as saw blades—the same type used in reciprocating saws. So with one tool, you can turn a screw as well as cut wood, drywall, and other household materials. It's available from a variety of manufacturers for $8 to $12.

3 TAPE MEASURE

No list of essential tools would be complete without a tape measure. "Whether you need to measure boxes for shipping gifts, drapes for your living room, or boards for hanging shelves, a tape measure is essential," says Don Vandervort, the author of more than 30 home improvement books and the founder of HomeTips.com. He recommends a 16-foot tape, which will range in price from $7 to $20, for most homeowners.

4 ADJUSTABLE RATCHET WRENCH

Securing nuts and driving bolts used to require a ratchet and entire toolbox of sockets. Now, Bennett says, manufacturers are making adjustable ratchet wrenches that can handle both tasks without all the assortment of parts. This tool costs around $20.

5 MULTI-TOOL

This collapsible handheld tool looks a lot like a Swiss Army knife, except it's outfitted with pliers, knives, screw-driving attachments, and other tools. In short, it has just about everything that you need for minor repairs. It's handy to take along when you travel, too; just be sure to pack it in your checked luggage and not in your carry-on. Depending on the brand and model, multi-tools can vary in price from $10 to over $100.

6 UTILITY KNIFE

For opening boxes and cutting insulation, matte board, and drywall, a basic utility knife equipped with a replaceable blade is indispensable. If you think you might take on more complex projects eventually, you may want to invest in a model that's outfitted with specialty blades for cutting roofing shingles and other materials, Vandervort says. Utility knives range in price from $5 to $25.

7 HAMMER

If you've browsed the tool display of your local hardware store or home center, you know that hammers come in all shapes and sizes. To help narrow your choices, Bennett recommends a finish hammer, which has a smooth face and a deeper hook that makes pulling out small nails easier. "For a long-lasting hammer, get one made from metal, with a rubber or metal handle," he adds. This should run you somewhere in the neighborhood of $5 to $25.

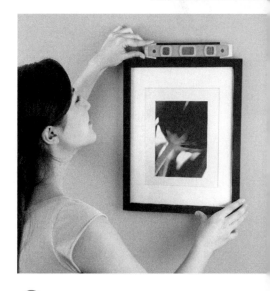

8 VISE GRIPS

Also known as locking pliers, vise grips provide holding power that you can't get from an ordinary wrench. "They're very handy to have around for jobs that require a second wrench or for spots in which an adjustable wrench will not work," Bennett says. Prices range from $5 to $30.

9 LEVEL

Nobody wants their prized artwork, photos, or flat-panel television hanging off-kilter, which is why a level rounds out our list of essential tools. And there's no reason to invest big bucks in a super-long level for everyday use. "An 8-inch torpedo level can help straighten pictures, shelves, appliances, and more," Vandervort says. Most 8-inch levels are in the $5 to $15 price range.

your list ——————

——————————
——————————
——————————
——————————
——————————

7 things never to leave home without

facts & figures

34

percent

The number of
Americans who don't
use all of their vacation
days, according to a
2009 survey by the
travel Web site
www.Expedia.com.

A VACATION MAY be just what the doctor ordered to break free from your daily routine and revitalize your body and brain. But getting there can be a headache all its own, especially if you realize in transit that you've forgotten something very, very important.

In most cases, you can pick up clothing and toiletries once you reach your destination. Travel documents, medications, and similar items can be much more difficult to replace—and trying to do so can wreak havoc on your time away.

Of course, you don't want to overpack, either, especially with increasingly stringent security and luggage guidelines. To help find the middle ground, we asked several travel experts what they make sure to stash in their bags when they're hitting the road for business or for pleasure. Keep their tips in mind for your next excursion.

1 SNACKS THAT PACK A PUNCH

Traveling can leave you without a proper meal for an extended period. To fend off hunger, take along a selection of ready-to-eat, healthy snacks. Energy bars, trail mix, and dried fruit are good, energizing choices, says Maurice A. Ramirez, PhD, founder and CEO of the consulting firm High Alert International and author of *The Complete Idiot's Guide to Disaster Preparedness.* Also put a couple of bottles of water in your checked bag or car.

2 THE RIGHT WARDROBE

Most people try to pack for every kind of weather and end up with a closet's worth of clothing in their suitcase. Ramirez recommends focusing on the essentials, which for him means having enough socks and underwear. Other items can be washed and worn again, but clean socks and underwear are the key to comfort. Other items on Ramirez's list include a jacket, a long-sleeve shirt, and a pair of pants—no matter how warm the destination may be. Also, pack a poncho for rain, a wide-brimmed hat for sun protection, and closed-toed shoes.

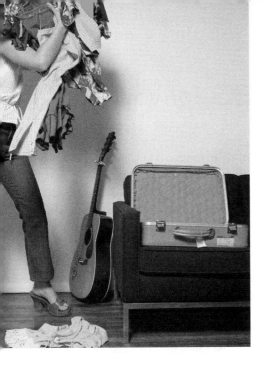

5 IMPORTANT PAPERS

Your driver's license and passport (when traveling internationally) are musts, as are your medical insurance cards and information, and credit cards. Also carry at least $150 in small bills, Ramirez says.

6 COMMUNICATION SUPPLIES

In addition to your cell phone charger, Paddock recommends picking up an extra cell phone battery for your trip, so you'll always have power. And take a roll of quarters for pay phones, just in case your cell phone doesn't work at all. Also handy: a list of information sources for your destination, including TV and radio stations, local access cable, local print media, weather services, and local government emergency operation center (EOC) numbers, Ramirez says.

7 THE COMFORTS OF HOME

The purpose of a vacation is relaxation, which is why Paddock includes certain items on her take-along list. "I always pack one change of clothing that will make me feel comfortable and cozy while I am away—usually a cashmere sweater and jeans in the winter and a comfy white shirt and white jeans in the summer," Paddock says. You might prefer a favorite tea, bath salts, a book or magazine, or a movie or TV show.

3 PERSONAL HYGIENE PRODUCTS

Many hotels provide soaps, shampoos, and other personal care items. But it's a good idea to take your own anyway, especially if you have sensitive skin that may not tolerate the product switch. Consider buying travel sizes of your favorite products. Also take along lip balm, sunscreen, insect repellant, toilet paper, and sanitary wipes, as you never know what conditions you might encounter on your trip.

4 THE PROPER PILLS

Prescription meds are a must, of course, but our experts also suggest several OTCs for extra insurance. Ramirez recommends a pain reliever such as Tylenol or Advil, as well as an anti-diarrheal medication, antacids, antihistamines, and decongestants. To this mix, Carolyn Paddock, a flight attendant for more than 20 years and author of the luxury travel blog www.InFlightInsider.com, adds a good multivitamin. It can help cover your nutritional bases while you're traveling.

your list

9 necessities for your car

mini LIST

Must-haves for winter driving

Winter travel presents its own set of hazards. If you must drive in winter weather, be sure to keep the following in your vehicle at all times.

1. **Ice scraper and brush.** Use the brush to clear accumulating snow from the roof, hood, and trunk of your car, as well as from the headlights and taillights.

2. **A small snow shovel.** Buy one that will fit into your trunk, advises Renee Grasso of Be Safe Plus, LLC.

3. **A hat, gloves, and a blanket.** Nobody wants to become stranded, but if you do, at least you'll be able to stay warm.

4. **Yaktrax.** These slip over your shoes to give you traction in even the most treacherous snow and ice.

NEXT TO OUR homes and workplaces, we probably spend more time in our cars than anywhere else. According to a 2009 survey of almost 2,000 people, the average American drives nearly 20 hours a week, logging over 200 miles in the process.

Considering the automobile's status as a "home away from home," it's understandable that we'd want our vehicles to have some of the same comforts to make those long commutes more bearable. We'd also like for them to deliver us to our destinations without a hitch, which means maintaining them properly and being prepared for roadside emergencies—whether a flat tire or something more serious.

With this wish list in mind, consider packing your trunk with the following tools and supplies for many miles of comfortable, safe, stress-free driving.

1 CLEANING SUPPLIES

Given the amount of time that you spend in your car, the interior is bound to get messy. With a small stash of cleaning supplies at the ready, you can wipe up your car—and yourself—before dirt and stains become a permanent part of your upholstery. Susan Foster, author of *Smart Packing for Today's Traveler,* recommends stocking your car with a travel-size box of tissues and hand wipes, antibacterial hand cleaner, a partial roll of paper towels, and a few trash bags (which you can tuck inside the paper towel roll for compact storage).

2 ROADSIDE VISIBILITY KIT

Such a kit can cost between $20 and $100, depending what's inside. It's a good investment. "The kit will help you stay visible to traffic in case you need to exit your car on the side of the road for any type of car trouble," says Renee Grasso of Be Safe Plus, LLC. Some kits contain a reflective triangle to set behind your vehicle and a vest to wear, while others offer more emergency roadside supplies.

3 CHARGERS

You never want your cell phone to die in a pinch, which is why Grasso recommends spending the extra dollars for a car charger whenever you buy a new cell phone. On the subject of charging, a set of jumper cables is a must-have, should you find yourself stranded with a dead battery.

4 A "LIFE HAMMER"

If your vehicle becomes submerged in water, you can use the hammer to break the side windows, Grasso says. It also will cut through a seatbelt, which can help free someone who's trapped.

5 SUSTENANCE

Packing a few healthy snacks like apples and nuts can nip hunger in the bud when you don't have time to stop for food. Carolyn Paddock, author of the travel blog InFlightInsider.com, carries along flavor packets to add to bottled water while she's driving.

6 A FIRST-AID KIT

Ideally you'll never need it, but if you do, you'll be glad to have one at the ready, says Maurice A. Ramirez, PhD. In addition to the usual first-aid supplies, Paddock suggests carrying Visine (for tired eyes) and individual packets of over-the-counter pain relievers and antacids.

7 A ROAD ATLAS

You may have made the switch to a GPS, but bear in mind that it can fail like any other electronic gadget. If it does, you'll be glad to have a road atlas as a backup. Buy the latest edition and stow it under your seat, just in case.

8 PERSONAL HYGIENE PRODUCTS

Especially after a long drive, you may want to freshen up before you exit your car. That's why Paddock keeps an "arrival kit" stocked with hand wipes, breath mints and gum, lip gloss, hair pins and ponytail holders, and a comb.

9 ORGANIZERS

Last but not least, you need a place to stow all of this stuff, so you can keep your car reasonably clutter-free. Myscha Theriault, a writer for the finance and frugal living blog WiseBread.com, recommends purchasing organizers that attach to your car seats. "The backs and sides of the front seats are seriously underutilized as storage space," she says. "Using organizers to hold things like maps, tissues, and first-aid and emergency supplies will help keep you sane."

your list

_____

_____

_____

_____

_____

_____

7 best excuses for calling in sick

facts & figures

20.7 million

The number of Americans who spend some time working from home, according to the Bureau of Labor Statistics.

THANKS TO THE arrival of H1N1, most of us are way more wary of the flu—and of those around us who seem to have symptoms. For better or worse, it's made taking an unplanned day off easier than ever. "You don't really need an excuse for calling in sick anymore," says Jim Joseph, president and partner of Lippe Taylor Brand Communications and author of *The Experience Effect*. "Gone are the days when you mustered through the flu and still went to work."

Clearly, you need to tread carefully when deciding whether to play hooky. But there are circumstances where it may be warranted. For example:

1 YOU'RE REALLY SICK

Going to work when you're coughing, aching, tired, and miserable is not good for anyone—especially not you. "Sleep, hydration, and more sleep help you kick a cold in one or two days, whereas going to work while you're sick may keep you from getting better for a week or more," says Ashley Koff, RD. "Your body can't focus on getting better and doing your 'other' job at the same time."

2 SOMEONE IN YOUR FAMILY IS SICK

If a family member requires immediate care, most employers will be understanding of that, says Roberta Matuson, author of *Tossed into Management!: The New Manager's Guide to Influencing Up and Down the Organization*. After all, most daycare facilities have guidelines that specifically prohibit bringing in children when they're sick.

3 YOU'RE FEELING BETTER

You still may be contagious, and it won't do your company much good if you show up and spread your germs to your co-workers. "Stay at home so that you don't infect everyone else!" Joseph says. Your doctor can tell you whether you're still infectious, so make an appointment.

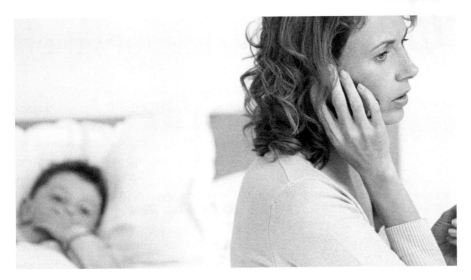

4 YOU NEED A MENTAL HEALTH DAY

Sometimes you just have to get away and clear your head. Tell your boss why you're taking off, though, so it doesn't come back to bite you. "And don't make a regular habit of it, or your employer may not take you seriously the next time you are truly sick," advises Peter Handal, CEO of Dale Carnegie Training.

5 YOU CAN WORK FROM HOME

Thanks to the Internet, cell phones, and even software that allows you to access your computer desktop offsite, "working from home" is easier than ever. So is playing hooky. "Now that I sign the checks, I don't believe in folks calling in sick," says Richard B. Chess, managing partner of Chess Law Firm. "But if they want to work from home on a laptop and make calls on their cell phones, it's acceptable to me. Packaging is everything!"

6 YOU NEED TO TEND TO A PERSONAL MATTER

Appointments and emergencies are a fact of life, and most employers will sign off on such absences as long as you don't take advantage. According to Matuson, the best excuses are car- or house-related, such as a stalled engine or a broken furnace.

7 YOU HAVE A JOB INTERVIEW

In this situation, you probably won't tell your boss the specifics of your absence (unless the two of you have a really good relationship). But if it's time to move on, career counselor Robin Ryan says do what you've got to do. "When you're preparing for a job interview and you need to review potential answers to the questions you'll likely be asked, then taking the day off to focus on this opportunity is a good idea," she says.

your list

_____

_____

_____

_____

_____

_____

8 easy ways to prevent identity theft

mini LIST

What to do if identify theft affects you

If you suspect that your identify has been stolen, Michael McCann, president of McCann Protective Services, recommends taking these actions without delay.

1. **Contact the fraud departments** of Equifax, Experian, and TransUnion and ask them to place a fraud alert on your accounts.

2. **Close the accounts** that you believe or know have been compromised.

3. **Contact the Social Security Administration** if you believe that your Social Security number has been compromised.

4. **Contact the US Postal Inspection Service** if you believe that your identity may have been compromised via the US mail system.

COMPUTERS HAVE SIMPLIFIED our lives in many ways. Unfortunately, this also holds true for criminals who make their livings by stealing our personal information and using it for their own gain.

Identity theft is real—and frightening. According to Michael McCann, president of McCann Protective Services in New York City and former security chief of the United Nations, nearly 8.4 million Americans became victims of identity theft in 2007, accumulating $49.3 billion in fraudulent charges. McCann describes identity theft as one of the fastest-growing crimes in the nation, accounting for as much as 25% of all annual losses because of credit card fraud.

There's much that we can do to safeguard our personal information and reduce the chances of it falling into the wrong hands. Among the most important and effective strategies are these.

1 SHRED, SHRED, SHRED!

Any documents that you wouldn't want a stranger to read should go into the shredder rather than the regular trash, advises Scott Stevenson, president and CEO of Eliminate ID Theft in Atlanta. This rule applies to any piece of unwanted paper that contains addresses, account numbers or access information, birthdates, driver's license numbers, employment information, envelopes and address labels, estimates, legal papers, luggage tags, medical information, passwords, report cards, signatures, Social Security numbers, transcripts, travel itineraries, and used airline tickets.

2 KEEP VITAL INFORMATION CLOSE

A thief needs just a few precious bits of your personal information to steal your identity. So be mindful of your driver's license, credit cards, and similar documents at all times, and especially when traveling, says Steven Domenikos, founder and CEO of IdentityTruth in Waltham, Massachusetts. Also, be careful with receipts. "Double-check credit card receipts when traveling out of the country, as some still print the cardholder's full name and credit card number," he says. "If you're going to throw receipts in the trash, be sure to shred them first."

3 OPT OUT

You can remove your name from the mailing lists for credit card and insurance offers by calling 1-888-5OPTOUT or visiting www.OptOutPrescreen.com. "In a few months, you'll notice a dramatic decrease in the amount of mail you receive," McCann says.

4 BE WARY OF ATMs

Most of us withdraw cash from our bank accounts via ATMs, but some of these machines are safer than others. "Only use ATMs with monitoring cameras, such as those in bank lobbies," Domenikos advises. "Avoid kiosk ATMs, as these freestanding units may not have cameras and are statistically more likely to be infected by skimmers (electronic devices that allow thieves to record account and PIN numbers)."

5 MAINTAIN SOME MYSTERY

If you're a fan of Facebook, MySpace, or Twitter, be careful about how much information you're divulging online. "These sites offer countless opportunities for identity theft," Domenikos says. "People should set restrictions on their profiles so that only friends can view their information." Domenikos also recommends deleting the Internet browser history and cookies if you're accessing these sites through public computers.

6 REVIEW STATEMENTS CAREFULLY

The best way to stay on top of suspicious credit card activity is to watch your statements like a hawk. If possible, check them online from a secure computer to make sure that nothing fishy is going on. "Also, monitor your credit report quar-

terly," McCann says. "The three major credit bureaus are Experian, Equifax, and Transunion. There are also reputable companies like Identity Guard that will monitor all of the major bureaus and provide joint reports for minimal fees."

7 ACT QUICKLY AFTER A DEATH

As appalling as it may seem, the deceased are frequent targets for identity theft. "Statistics show that identity thieves prey on the sick or deceased—a practice known as ghosting—due to an increased likelihood that the theft will go unde-tected," Domenikos says. He recommends contacting the Social Security Administra-tion, notifying credit reporting agencies, and closing all accounts in the deceased person's name.

8 TRY A MONITORING SERVICE

Considering the ever-growing risk of identity theft, signing up with a reputable monitoring service might be a good idea. "These services provide alerts beyond what shows up on your credit report," Domenikos says. When choosing a service, he adds, comparison shop to find one that provides the greatest value. To make sure you end up with a monitoring service you can trust, you may want to ask your banker or financial advisor if they have any recommendations. There is a fee involved with most of these services.

your list

7 ways to cheer yourself up

my favorite...
Fix for a Bad Mood

John M. Rowley, director of fitness and wellness at the American Institute of Healthcare & Fitness in Raleigh, North Carolina

Rowley is a firm believer in the power of laughter to lift a bad mood. "Many years ago, my wife and I lost everything in a business deal. We had two babies with a third on the way, and life was hard," he recalls. "My wife had an old record of Steve Martin, and we would listen to it and laugh until we cried." Rowley credits his wife's wisdom—and Martin's "wild and crazy" antics—with helping them not only to bounce back but to eventually recapture their success.

ANY NUMBER OF things can send you into a funk—your job, the weather, an unexpected bill. When it happens, you just might want to settle in for a good sulk. And that's totally ok in certain circumstances. But there will be times when you need to shake off your bad mood, and quick. Otherwise, you may not be as focused and productive as you'd like.

How you go about snapping out of a snit really depends on what works for you. Experiment with these tips from our experts.

1 SET A TIME LIMIT

You can let your doldrums run their course—but give them a deadline. "For example, you might tell yourself that you're going to feel down for about 15 minutes. Then you're going to pull yourself together and do something that you really enjoy," says Rallie McAllister, MD, MPH. The idea is to not let your bad mood consume you so that you can't see anything but the downside of the situation.

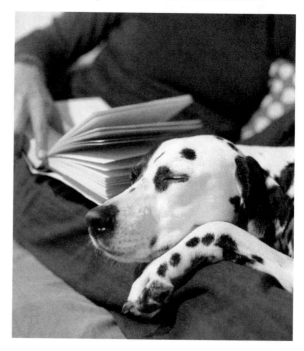

2 THINK POSITIVELY

When you're ready, you can begin to bounce back from your bad mood by considering all that's right and good in your life, says Janie Harden Fritz, PhD, professor of communications and rhetorical studies at Duquesne University in Pittsburgh. "Focus your attention on what you have, what is possible, and what your next step might be in terms of the situation that you find yourself in," she suggests. "Identifying positive action provides a sense of self-efficacy, or 'I can do this.' Taking one successful step forward leads to another."

3 MAKE A LIST

It might help to write down all of the things that you're grateful for, that you think are going well, and that you're looking forward to. "This helps provide perspective," McAllister says. "Chances are the problem you're facing will look rather insignificant when compared to all of the great things in your life."

4 DO SOMETHING YOU LOVE

Whether it's taking a walk, spending time on a hobby, or spending the day at the beach, you need to allow time for yourself. "It's all about focus of attention," Fritz says. "When you're sad, you need periods of time to think constructively and move forward."

5 VOLUNTEER

Helping others never fails to lift the spirits. It allows us to feel useful and purposeful. "It also gives us reason to feel appreciative for all the wonderful things in our own lives," McAllister notes.

6 FIND A FURRY FRIEND

Sometimes a good cuddle with Fido or Fluffy is all that's needed to put us in the right frame of mind. "Animals have a way of cheering us up and making us feel better," McAllister says. If you don't have a pet, she recommends that you try volunteering at an animal shelter. "That way, you'll get all of the benefits of interacting with pets and volunteering in one fell swoop," she says.

7 CHEER UP SOMEONE ELSE!

By shifting your attention to another person, you may help yourself in the process. "It redirects your emotional energy in constructive ways and starves out self-pity," Fritz says.

your list

6 ways to cheer up someone else

my favorite . . .
Way to Cheer Someone

Janie Harden Fritz, PhD, professor at Duquesne University in Pittsburgh

As painful as it is to see someone we care about in despair, trying to force a joyful, positive attitude on the person is not helpful. "I refuse to offer false comfort with comments such as 'Everything's okay' or 'Don't worry about it—it's no great loss anyway,'" Fritz says. "It's important to embrace the reality of sadness and loss, and it's okay not to feel great all the time."

True cheer comes from taking stock of the real, Fritz adds. "When we acknowledge our emotions, we can let them have their place and then find a way to the authentic cheerfulness that comes from dealing with circumstances in constructive ways," she says.

THINK FOR A moment about the last time someone came to you with a personal problem and in need of an emotional boost. Did you give the person an automatic "Things will be fine?" Or did you clam up and say nothing, for fear you might make matters worse?

Both responses are completely natural. But if you put yourself in that person's shoes for a moment, you can see how neither would have been especially helpful. A better choice may be to ask, "What can I do to help?" offers Rallie McAllister, MD, MPH. Sometimes just showing concern and being willing to lend an ear (or a shoulder) is enough to cheer a person. These tips can help, too.

1 REMIND THEM THAT THEY MATTER
As you may know from personal experience, when you're in a funk, you can feel as though no one cares about you or understands you. So one of the best things you can do for someone in a similar circumstance is to let the person know that he or she is important to you and that you want him or her to be okay.

2 OFFER A COMPLIMENT
A little kick in the self-esteem can lift the spirits of just about anyone. Tell someone that you admire her cooking skills, that he's a terrific father/son/brother, that no one can match her organizational skills or knack for giving a presentation. "Recognize what the person does really well, and express your opinion," McAllister says.

3 GIVE A HUG
This advice depends on how well you know the other person and whether this type of contact is appropriate for the two of you. But as McAllister explains, hugging feels good for a reason, and it has to do with human chemistry. "Warm, loving physical contact triggers the release of oxytocin, a hormone and neurotransmitter that creates a sense of bonding and other positive feelings," McAllister says. "Nothing elicits a positive response as immediately and completely as a good hug."

4 JUST LISTEN

When you are the friend offering a shoulder to lean on, keep your role in the proper perspective. Often that shoulder is all the person is looking for—not advice or a pep talk. "Sometimes people need to express their feelings and need to know that they're being heard," McAllister says. "Remember, you don't need to have a solution. For the other person, just being able to air the problem to a sympathetic listener can be remarkably therapeutic and healing."

5 EMPHASIZE THE POSITIVE

While it's okay for the two of you to spend some time together down in the dumps, at some point you should make attempt to steer the person toward a more positive frame of mind, says Janie Harden Fritz, PhD, professor at Duquesne University in Pittsburgh. Don't rush it, of course, but recognize when your friend or loved one may need a push to move on. Otherwise, all that wallowing will turn counterproductive.

6 END ON A HIGH NOTE

Not every attempt to cheer someone is going to be successful. Sometimes a person just wants to be miserable, and you may need to move on, for your own sanity. Whatever transpires, try to end the exchange with the other person by being upbeat, advises Shoshana Bennett, PhD, an expert on postpartum depression and an author of several books on the topic. She suggests listening and validating for as long as you feel is appropriate. Then close the conversation by reminding the person that whatever is going on will pass, that he or she will survive it, and that you're there to help.

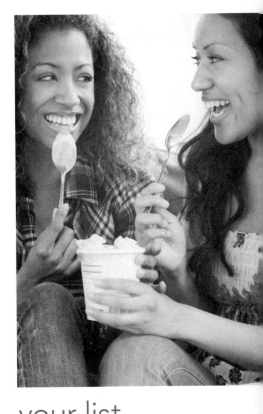

your list

_____
_____
_____
_____
_____
_____
_____
_____
_____
_____
_____
_____
_____

7 top tunes to move you

mini LIST

Perfect playlists

Tom Moon, a music contributor to National Public Radio and the author of *1,000 Recordings to Hear Before You Die,* has compiled playlists for just about every occasion. Here's just a sampling of his recommendations:

HITTING THE ROAD:

1. **The Allman Bros. Band:** Anything from *Live at the Fillmore East*

2. **Bob Seger:** "Turn The Page" from *Greatest Hits Vol. 1*

ENTERTAINING GUESTS:

1. **James Brown:** The entire album *Sex Machine*

2. **Tito Puente and his Orchestra:** "Llego Mijon," from *Dance Mania*

CLEANING HOUSE:

1. **Bob Marley and the Wailers:** "Three Little Birds" from *Exodus*

2. **Aretha Franklin:** "Do Right Woman" from *I Never Loved a Man the Way I Love You*

WE DON'T NEED research to tell us that music makes us feel good. We just have to slip in a CD or put on our headphones. In an instant, we're transported to another place where we can relax, focus, or be inspired.

Recently, though, scientists have been uncovering evidence that turning on the tunes has a very real, positive impact on our minds and bodies. Music therapy is an entire discipline devoted to understanding and using music's healing power to alleviate stress, manage pain, and promote wellness in other ways.

Our motivation for listening may be driven by something more basic: It can make something that isn't necessarily enjoyable—like exercising or housecleaning—a lot more pleasant. And time seems to fly by when we're plugged in to our iPods.

With this in mind, we asked our experts to identify the best musical genres to complement certain tasks. Some went a step further, suggesting particular artists and tunes for your playlist. So listen up!

1 BEST TUNES TO . . . START YOUR DAY

Rhonda M. Johnson, MD, MPH, medical director of health equity and quality services for Highmark, Inc., in Pittsburgh, likes to listen to gospel and inspirational music first thing in the morning. "Many researchers believe that there is a scientific correlation between faith, spirituality, and health. Personally, I believe that the body, soul, and spirit work together in an interconnected way," she says. Her favorite recording artist: Yolanda Adams.

2 BEST TUNES TO . . . CRAM FOR AN EXAM

Whether you're studying for a big test or just trying to focus carefully on what you're reading, David L. Katz, MD, MPH, suggests classical or spa music. "Studies suggest a calming, concentrating effect," he says. "Bach may be best of all, thanks to the mathematical precision of his composition."

3 BEST TUNES TO . . . WARM UP

Remember that the purpose of warming up is to prime your muscles for physical activity. So you want songs that have a more modest tempo. "We know that walkers, runners, and cyclists often match their pace to the beat of the music," says Stacey Rosenfeld, PhD, a sports psychologist and an expert in the treatment of eating disorders and body image issues. "So for a warm-up, keep your tunes relatively tame." Her suggestions: "California" by Phantom Planet and "Make Me Believe" by Angel Taylor.

4 BEST TUNES TO . . . GO WALKING

According to Rosenfeld, tunes with a tempo of at least 120 beats per minute (bpm) are ideal for walkers. She also recommends songs with lyrics that mirror your activity, so for a walking workout, for example, you might load your iPod with "Walking on Sunshine" (Katrina and the Waves) and "Walk this Way" (Run-DMC). Going for a run? Listen to "I Ran So Far Away" (Flock of Seagulls) and "Running Down a Dream" (Tom Petty).

5 BEST TUNES TO . . . COOL DOWN

For the last few minutes of your workout, you should be scaling back your intensity and allowing your heartbeat to return to normal. Music can help here, too. Choose songs that have fewer beats per minute (around 120 or fewer) and that give you props for what you've just accomplished. "I like 'The World's Greatest' by R. Kelly, 'Pride' by Syntax, and 'First Day of My Life' by Bright Eyes," Rosenfeld says.

6 BEST TUNES TO . . . CLEAN YOUR HOUSE

They're called chores for a reason: For most of us, doing them feels like drudgery.

But that doesn't mean you can't have a little fun with them. Turning on the tunes makes them go that much faster. "I find that music from the 1970s is good for chores that you've been putting off," says Bob Mamet, an internationally acclaimed jazz pianist and composer in Venice Beach, California. "For some reason, hearing Hall and Oates or Earth, Wind, and Fire makes people want to clean the basement! I think it's because the '70s were a carefree decade, with carefree music."

7 BEST TUNES TO . . . RELAX

This is really a matter of personal preference, although Mamet has a strong candidate that almost anybody will enjoy. "I've found that perhaps the most relaxing album of all time is *Kind of Blue* by Miles Davis," he says. "Even those unfamiliar with jazz find that it soothes them, while at the same time giving them a psychological and cerebral lift."

your list

_____

_____

_____

_____

_____

_____

_____

_____

_____

_____

_____

_____

_____

_____

_____

9 simple ways to repair the world

my favorite ...
Anecdote

Kathy LeMay, founder, president, and CEO of Raising Change

Celebrities and billionaires have a lot of money to give away. We read about it all the time: big names, big causes, and big wallets. "But here's a secret: Celebrities and billionaires won't change the world," LeMay says. "You will."

How? Teddy Roosevelt said it best: by "doing what you can, with what you have, where you are."

"When each of us gives our money, time, and skills, it's real philanthropy in action," LeMay says. "This is the tipping point that will change the world for the better."

IN A WORLD where so much seems beyond our control, it's easy to sink into cynicism and apathy. Yes, we can offer our skills and resources to help improve others' lives, as well as our own. But really, how much of a difference can any one of us really make?

Quite a lot, as it turns out. When each of us does his or her part, the sum of our efforts can lift all of us and bring about positive change.

But we needn't wait for the next disaster to contribute to our community. "Little things, when done by many people on a daily basis, can make the world a better place over time," says Peter Handal, CEO of Dale Carnegie Training.

Ready to give back, but not sure where to begin? Consider these ideas from our experts.

1 GIVE WHAT YOU CAN
Even in these cash-strapped times, every one of us has something to offer—whether it's dollars, or manpower, or personal connections. "Helping those who are less fortunate is one of the easiest and most meaningful ways to contribute to the greater good," Handal says.

2 GO ALL OUT
Once you commit to something, always give 110%, Handal adds. The person who does this—and who doesn't let fear of failure discourage or disrupt his or her efforts—is the one who ultimately succeeds. Look at it this way: Every nonprofit organization that exists today grew from one person's vision and determination to bring it to fruition.

3 TEACH A CHILD
By passing on your knowledge to the next generation, you are improving the world in the long run. "Teach children about ways to contribute to the world through philanthropy and volunteer service," suggests Gail Bower, president of Bower & Company Consulting in Philadelphia. "Help them to cultivate their passion for meaningful organizations that are getting results."

4 BE HAPPY

Spreading joy to others is as noble as any mission to make the world a better place. "Taking time to acknowledge the people and things that define your world, and expressing your care and compassion for them, creates a positive energy that others will want to embrace and share," Handal says.

5 LIVE VICARIOUSLY THROUGH OTHERS

Expressing genuine joy at the accomplishments of others will spread goodwill. "Our sense of worth thrives on communicative nourishment," notes Janie Harden Fritz, PhD. "Provide nourishment for someone else, even if you've not received it. By making things better for others, you encourage yourself, too."

6 TEXT LESS, TALK MORE

"I find that when people sit down and talk to each other, problems tend to get resolved much faster and easier, and in a way that meets everyone's needs," says Jim Joseph, author of *The Experience Effect.* "The trouble is that people don't talk directly about issues, so the issues just get bigger." His advice: Shut down your laptop, hang up your cell phone, and have a conversation face-to-face.

7 SNEAK IN SOME NICENESS

If you're nice on the sly, it does good in two ways: You've done a good deed, and you've done it in a way that requires no acknowledgment. "Do something nice for someone every day and don't get found out . . . ever!" urges Jean Kelley, president and founder of Jean Kelley Leadership Consulting and author of *Get a Job, Keep a Job.*

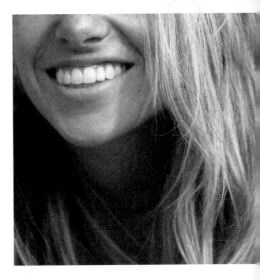

8 RESPECT OTHERS . . . ALWAYS

Ultimately, making the world a better place is about respecting those with whom we share it, regardless of what they're able to bring to the table. "Remember that the other guy is a human being, too, and probably prefers love to war when given a chance," says David L. Katz, MD, MPH.

9 SMILE MORE

Our final suggestion for changing the world is also the simplest. "A smile is free, it's easy, and it has wonderfully positive effect on others," Handal says. "It's contagious!"

your list ———

———

———

———

———

———

9 lessons to change your life

my favorite . . .
Strategy for Loving Life

Larry Valant, author of *Stop Breaking the Rules*

Valant says that one of the hardest lessons he ever had to learn was that he actually controlled very little in his life. "Because I thought I had much greater control than I did, I worked very hard to make everything and everyone behave 'correctly,'" he recalls. Eventually, Valant realized that most of his stress was being driven by his efforts to control situations—and people—that he really couldn't. "Once I made this discovery, I tried focusing on those things that I could control (my own thoughts and actions) and letting go of those things I couldn't (just about everything else)," he says. "This epiphany was the beginning of my ability to truly enjoy life."

THE PURSUIT OF happiness is so important that our Founding Fathers wrote it into the Constitution. We take this right very seriously, and when it eludes us, we can't experience life fully. "Life is supposed to be happy," notes Jim Joseph, author of *The Experience Effect*. "When it isn't, you need to make a change."

This is an important point: For your emotional and physical well-being, your happiness ought to be a priority for you. "Too many of us put happiness on the back burner in favor of doing more. But often we end up with less," says Michele Jewett, founder of Michele J Coaching in San Diego. "Studies show that you will be healthier and have access to a higher level of thinking when you are in your 'happy zone.'"

Here's how to translate your passion into your personal rules to live by.

1 DO WHAT YOU LOVE

You spend too much of your life at work to be doing something that you aren't truly passionate about. And if your heart isn't in your job anymore, you may need to think about moving on. "Research has found that people who love their work take 25% fewer sick or personal days," says Debra Condren, PhD, founder of Manhattan Business Coaching and author of *Ambition Is Not a Dirty Word*. "To live a rewarding life, follow your most ambitious dreams and always strive to do meaningful, challenging, inspiring work that uses your talents and pays you what you're worth."

2 BE HONEST

No good ever comes from lying, even the little white variety. "By hiding the truth and covering up failures, we only deceive ourselves. The truth always becomes known," says Larry Valant, president of the Valant and Company consulting firm in Colorado and author of *Stop Breaking the Rules*. "A reputation as a truth-teller is the foundation for building self-respect and winning others' admiration."

3 SEE AMBITION AS A VIRTUE

Ambition should not be viewed as vain or selfish. It is an asset to be cultivated. "Being the happiest person that you can possibly be comes from always staying true to your ambition rather than giving in to social duress to put it after every other priority in your life," Condren says.

4 REACH OUT EVERY DAY

Whether it's to volunteer or to maintain your social circle, making a commitment to staying in touch with those around you is vital to your happiness. "I try to reach out to someone every day," says Richard B. Chess, managing partner of Chess Law Firm. "Everyone needs help, and they are just waiting for someone to care."

5 TREAT YOUR BODY WITH RESPECT

Remember that everything you put in your body has an effect on your health. So strive to make health-conscious choices like organic whole foods instead of processed foods. "When we make deliberate choices about what we eat and drink, we feel empowered as opposed to deprived," says Ashley Koff, RD.

6 STOP SAYING "SHOULD"

If you keep thinking that you "should" be doing something, there's probably a reason that you aren't doing it! "Take all of the 'should's' off your list unless you can truly turn them into 'want-to's,'" Jewett says.

7 NEVER STOP LEARNING

No matter how small the lesson, the key to continued growth is to try to learn something new every day. "Carl Jung said that we have the capacity to continue to grow and to deepen our self-awareness and consciousness until the day we die," Condren notes. "What better way to live an inspired, fulfilling life than to stay dedicated to self-actualization?"

8 REMEMBER: TO ERR IS HUMAN

Everyone makes mistakes; the trick is to not make the same one twice. When you learn from it, you grow. "You can't change a mistake, but you can change its effect on you," says Janie Harden Fritz, PhD.

9 LIVE FOR TODAY

Along the same line, obsessing about what happened in the past or what might happen in the future undermines your happiness in the present. "I have counseled clients who are going through such difficult situations that their fears overwhelm them," Valant says. "My advice to them: 'Stay in today! Focus on what you can do today!'" This in-the-moment approach has helped Valant and his clients weather the most challenging times—and it's helped them rediscover their true happiness along the way.

your list

index

Underscored page references indicate boxed text.